The Health Information Exchange Formation Guide

The Authoritative Guide for Planning and Forming an HIE in Your State, Region, or Community

Laura Kolkman, RN, MS, FHIMSS

Bob Brown

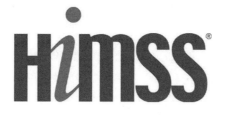

HIMSS Mission

To lead healthcare transformation through the effective use of health information technology.

Printed in the U.S.A. 5 4 3 2 1

Requests for permission to reproduce any part of this work should be sent to:

Permissions Editor
HIMSS
230 E. Ohio St., Suite 500
Chicago, IL 60611-3270
cmclean@himss.org

ISBN: 978-0-9821070-8-9

The inclusion of an organization name, product or service in this publication should not be construed as an endorsement of such organization, product or service, nor is the failure to include an organization name, product or service to be construed as disapproval.

For more information about HIMSS, please visit www.himss.org.

About the Authors

Laura Kolkman, RN, MS, FHIMSS
President
Mosaica Partners, LLC

Laura Kolkman has more than three decades of experience in healthcare, information technology, and consulting. She began her professional career as a registered nurse, spending ten years in various clinical positions including staff nurse, nurse manager, nursing instructor, and assistant director of nursing. At that point, intrigued by the potential for using information technology to improve healthcare quality, she returned to school and earned a master's degree in computer science.

After receiving her graduate degree Ms. Kolkman's career advanced rapidly as she held a number of increasingly important management and IT-related positions. At a Fortune 50 global pharmaceutical firm, she was responsible for IT strategy, applications development and delivery, systems validation, and regulatory compliance in support of the firm's global R&D division. In that role, she managed a staff of professionals located in the U.S., Europe, and Asia.

Ms. Kolkman also served as vice president and chief information officer for a $1.5 billion national pharmacy services provider where, as CIO, she was responsible for the development, implementation, and management of the firm's IT and associated resources.

In 2005, Ms. Kolkman established Mosaica Partners. The firm quickly earned a national reputation as specialists in health information exchange. The company provides a wide range of consulting services to its clients that relate to the planning, formation, operation, and optimization of health information exchanges (HIEs) and the optimization of healthcare informatics-based business process. In addition, the firm provides advice and counsel to HIE/HIT vendors with an interest in entering—or enhancing their position—in the health information marketplace.

Ms. Kolkman is an active supporter of the health information exchange movement. She was the FY 08-09 Chair of the Health Information Exchange Steering Committee of HIMSS where, among other duties, she was actively involved in preparing the HIMSS briefing paper on the subject of health information for the (then) incoming administration of President Barack Obama. She is often invited to speak at industry conferences and is frequently quoted in the press about trends and developments in HIE. She has published many articles on subjects related to health information exchange and was a contributor to the *Guide to Establishing a Regional Health Information Organization*, published by HIMSS in 2007.

Ms. Kolkman holds an MS in Computer Science from Western Michigan University and a BSN from the University of Michigan, where she graduated Summa Cum Laude.

Bob Brown
Vice President, Professional Services
Mosaica Partners, LLC

Bob Brown is an internationally recognized authority on consulting and the consulting process. His well-rounded background includes accomplishments in developing and delivering consulting service offerings, developing consulting methods and tools, and product management of both financial services and technology products. He has additional management and technical level experience in publishing, telecommunications, and information systems.

In 2008, Mr. Brown joined Mosaica Partners as an advisor and consultant in the areas of business and consulting practices. He led the team that developed Mosaica's HIE Maturity Framework, and HIE formation methodology, on which this book is based. In his present position, he oversees the delivery of all of Mosaica's consulting and advisory services, often participating in engagements in the role of executive consultant or methodology exponent. He is currently focusing on the establishment of Mosaica Research, an affiliate firm that will provide market intelligence services to HIE/HIT vendors.

In addition to his work at Mosaica Partners, from 2004 to 2010 Mr. Brown held the position of Managing Director of Consulting Intelligence, a specialized consulting practice which he established in 2004. Consulting Intelligence advised clients in the areas of sourcing, selecting, utilizing, and managing consulting firms and consulting projects.

Previously, Mr. Brown was a senior consultant and subject matter professional with IBM Business Consulting Services and a member of their Customer Relationship Management (CRM) Strategy Practice. He specialized in developing, deploying and implementing CRM strategies that were designed to help IBM's clients transform their organizations to efficiently, effectively, and profitably deliver appropriate value-based experiences to their customers. Mr. Brown also taught consulting practices and methodology at IBM Executive Consulting Institute locations in Europe, North America, and Asia. One of his last assignments at IBM was Resident CRM Subject Matter Professional at IBM's North American Strategic Envisioning Center.

Prior to IBM, Mr. Brown held management and technical positions with the Bank of Hawaii, Pacific TeleCommunications Council, VeriFone, and The Direct Connection Co., Inc.

Acknowledgments

We have many people to thank for their contributions to this book. First and foremost, we'd like to thank the publications group at HIMSS for making it possible to share our research on and experience with HIEs at this extraordinary point in time.

We'd like to thank those who worked with us in putting the book together, providing input, reviewing content, and in so many ways, supporting us. Coordinating it all was Fran Rubino, Laura's assistant, who kept everything well organized through all the brainstorming sessions, heated discussions, and final preparation. Without her gentle prodding and quiet efficiency, we could not have completed this book.

We'd also like to thank Fran Perveiler, our editor, and Pam Matthews, both at HIMSS, for their enthusiasm for reviewing manuscripts, insightful input, and patience with us as we went through many iterations of construct and content.

Special thanks goes to those who rolled up their sleeves and reviewed specific sections of the book: Gerry Hinkley, JD (Co-Chair, Health Care Industry Team, Pillsbury Winthrop Shaw Pittman LLP), Jennifer Breuer, JD (Partner, Drinker Biddle & Reath), and Lisa Gallagher (HIMSS) who all provided insight into the privacy section, Dave Minch (HIPAA/HIE Project Manager, John Muir Health) and Mark Jacobs (Director of Technology Services, Wellspan Health) who contributed to the technology and security sections, Richard Soley (CEO, Object Management Group) for his insights on standards, Mark Haas for his review of the governance section, Mary Ellen Myers for her always excellent research, Barbara Bateman for her insights and review, and Robyn Winters for her help in casting the story.

Interviewees

We offer our sincere thanks and appreciation to our friends and colleagues listed below. They freely gave not only their time, but also their wisdom by sharing their experiences with us so that we could share them with you.

Laura L. Adams
President & CEO, Rhode Island Quality
    Institute
Faculty, Institute for Healthcare
    Improvement
Board Chair, National eHealth
    Collaborative

Holt Andersen
Executive Director
North Carolina Healthcare Information
    and Communications Alliance
    (NCHICA)

Deb Bass
Executive Director
Nebraska Health Information Initiative
    (NeHII)

Larry Biggio
Executive Director
Wyoming Health Information
    Organization

Jeffrey S. Blair, MBA
Director of Health Informatics
LCF Research, New Mexico Health
    Information Collaborative (NMHIC)

Devore S. Culver, MM
Executive Director and CEO
HealthInfoNet, Maine

Didi Davis
President/Principal
Serendipity Health, LLC, Tennessee

Joy Duling, MSW
Project Director for HIE & Regional
    Extension Center
Quality Quest for Health of Illinois

Carladenise Edwards
HIT Coordinator*
State of Georgia

Helen L. Hill, FHIMSS
Chair, Southeast Michigan Health
    Information Exchange (SEMHIE)
Technical/Functional Work Group
Director, IT Consulting and HIE,
    Henry Ford Health System – CSC

Mark J. Jacobs, MHA, CPHIMS,
    FHIMSS
Director of Technology Services
Wellspan Health, Pennsylvania

Liesa Jenkins
Executive Director*
CareSpark, Tennessee

David L. Johnson
President and CEO
BioCrossroads, Indiana

John P. Kansky, MSE, MBA, CPHIMS,
    FHIMSS
Vice President - Business Development
Indiana Health Information Exchange
    (IHIE)

Ted Kremer
Executive Director
Rochester RHIO, New York

Philip W. Magistro
Deputy Director, Program
    Implementation
State Government HIT Coordinator,
    Pennsylvania

Michael Matthews, MSPH
CEO
MedVirginia

Trudi L. Matthews
Director of Policy and Public Relations
HealthBridge, Ohio

David A. Minch
Security Committee Co-Chair,
California Privacy & Security Advisory
    Board
HIPAA/HIE Project Manager
John Muir Health

Beth Nagel
Health Information Technology
    Coordinator
Michigan Department of Community
    Health

* Position at time of interview

Gina Bianco Perez, MPA
President, Advances in Management,
    Inc.
Executive Director, Delaware Health
    Information Network (DHIN)

Christopher B. Sullivan, PhD
Administrator
Office of Health Information Exchange
Florida Center for Health Information
    and Policy Analysis
Agency for Health Care Administration

Dick Thompson
Executive Director/CEO
Quality Health Network, Colorado

Brad Tritle, CIPP
Executive Director*
Arizona Health-e Connection

Andrew Weniger
Program Manager
North Carolina Healthcare Information
    and Communications Alliance
    (NCHICA)

---

* Position at time of interview

Preface

As W. Edwards Deming once said, "It is not necessary to change. Survival is not mandatory." For us, however, significant and timely change *is* mandatory if the healthcare delivery system in this country is to survive in any reasonable form.

Viewed from an international perspective, America spends more money, per capita, on healthcare than any other country on the planet. From a practical perspective, reducing the alarmingly high—and continually growing—cost of providing our healthcare is essential. Why? If left unchecked, and continuing at its current rate, our growing outlay for healthcare could literally bankrupt this country.

At the same time, compared to other developed countries the U.S. ranks abysmally low in the quality of healthcare that's actually being delivered. From an economic perspective, our antiquated approach to managing health information on paper and in silos introduces significant and unnecessary inefficiency into our healthcare delivery system. The result is a hidden 'inefficiency tax' that each one of us pays in the form of higher insurance premiums and direct payments for services.

Clearly, something is wrong. Especially when you realize that a leading cause of both of these problems are the hundreds and thousands of antiquated, paper-based systems still in use today to capture, store, and move our medical records—preventing us from providing the quality of care that we are capable of providing. Transitioning from paper to electronic records and sharing information electronically has already been accomplished in other industries. Extraordinary efficiencies and process improvements have been realized. Now it's time to do the same in healthcare.

Fortunately, a lot of people agree on this point. And the timing couldn't be better. A window of opportunity has opened. The federal government recently introduced programs that will allocate billions of dollars for the transition of health records to an electronic format and making that information sharable electronically. Each of the states and U.S. territories is also actively involved as a result of the availability of those federal funds. Different states and territories are taking different approaches, but they're all involved in doing their part to enable this essential transition.

At the regional or community level, people from all walks of life are coming together to talk about the best way to make electronic health information readily available in their area. These conversations have been taking place for the past 20 years or more, but until the recent and massive infusion of federal funds, the effort required to build the critical mass necessary to actually form and operate a state, regional or community health information exchange organization was often too difficult to muster.

Given this new opportunity, now is the time for states, regions, and communities to come together to enable this transition and to begin to realize the many benefits that the movement to electronic sharing of health information will make possible.

We believe this capability—being able to capture, store, and move our personal health records electronically—is an essential enabler that, when properly implemented, will positively improve the quality of healthcare in this country. Not only will it improve the overall efficiency of the healthcare delivery process, it will lead directly to improved patient outcomes and will be a significant influence on lowering the high costs currently associated with delivering healthcare.

This book provides you with a practical, step-by-step approach to forming a health information exchange in your state, region, or community. Based on extensive research and our own direct experience as HIE consultants, we describe a structured approach to forming a health information exchange organization, one that incorporates leading practices that have helped other organizations as they journeyed through the planning and formation stages and then moved on to successful operations.

We begin the book by giving you a high-level overview of health information exchange, followed by a brief discussion of why we believe it's important. We then describe the essential steps involved in planning and forming a health information exchange. To help you on your journey, we include examples, checklists, and end of chapter references.

As an added benefit, HIMSS is making many of the checklists and the end of chapter reference links available on a companion website. **Visit www.himss.org/ hieformationguide.**

Forming a Health Information Exchange is a journey.
This book provides you with the right tools and points you in the right direction.
But only you, and your stakeholders, can take the actual steps necessary to
successfully form and operate an HIE.

We hope this book is a valuable resource in helping you understand the subject of health information exchange and—if you are directly involved in planning and forming such an organization—a handy source of practical advice and specific techniques to ease your journey. Others have successfully made this journey. You can too!

Laura Kolkman
Bob Brown

Contents

CHAPTER 1

The HIE Landscape

"...We can envision a transformation of our health system to improve health care quality, efficiency, equity, and safety through the use of health information technology..."

David Blumenthal, MD, MPP
National Coordinator for Health Information Technology

INTRODUCTION

You are about to embark on one of the most important and exciting journeys of your life. Creating the capabilities required to enable electronic health information exchange (HIE) is a journey of change that holds the promise of better healthcare for all of us. We are now seeing unprecedented amounts of attention, resources, and real money beginning to be allocated to this cause. There are major efforts at the national and state levels and in many individual regions. This convergence of attention, resources, and funding has created a once-in-a-generation opportunity and has spawned what we view as a major societal movement.

Before you begin any journey—especially one going into uncharted territory like HIE—it is always wise to arm yourself with a good understanding of the landscape. And HIE is a landscape that is undergoing a seismic shift.

We begin this chapter, and this book, with a brief history of HIE in the U.S. and an overview of the current HIE landscape—as of the writing of this book in late 2010. It is important for you to understand this landscape as you begin your HIE formation efforts and therefore need the ability to educate your stakeholders and the community at large about the value of HIEs. We provide a briefing on the context within which HIE is taking place in the U.S., identify and describe key federal agencies and initiatives, and provide a broad list of online resources.

The discussion in this chapter is meant as an overview to ensure that you are aware of the key organizations, programs, and potential funding sources that could impact your efforts to form an HIE. References are provided at the end of chapters that you can use to gain more in-depth information on the topics presented. Because the HIE landscape continues to change at a rapid pace, we encourage you to frequently check those online resources listed in the references to ensure you have the most current information.

First, we concentrate on the initiatives at the federal level and then discuss how these will impact you at the state, regional, and community levels. As we write this, virtually every state is in the process of developing or implementing its HIE strategic and operational plan. While we do not discuss the specifics of each state's plan, we do provide the basics that each of the states are required to address to receive its share of the HIE-related American Recovery and Reinvestment Act of 2009 (ARRA) funding. We spend more time discussing the roles of the state HIE efforts and the regional extension centers in this chapter than some of the other initiatives. This is because they directly impact much of what you need to accomplish and can serve as good resources.

WHAT IS HEALTH INFORMATION EXCHANGE?

The *HIMSS Dictionary of Healthcare Information Technology Terms, Acronyms, and Organizations*[1] defines health information exchange (HIE) as:

1. The sharing action between any two or more organizations with an executed business/legal arrangement that have deployed commonly agreed-upon technology with applied standards, for the purpose of electronically exchanging health-related data between the organizations; and

2. A catchall phrase for all health information exchanges, including regional health information organizations (RHIOs), state level health information exchanges (SLHIEs), health information organizations (HIOs), Agency for Healthcare Research and Quality (AHRQ)-funded communities, and private exchanges.

In this book, we use HIE to refer to both the exchange of health information, as well as the organization that supports the exchange.

THE FOUNDATIONAL ORGANIZATIONS

What we regard as the current era of HIE began in earnest in 2004. Prior to that time—going back to the 1990s and earlier—some very forward thinking individuals and communities began community health information networks, or, as they are commonly called, CHINs. Most of these early efforts did not succeed. However, there are some that have endured—or spawned successful efforts that are in operation today, such as the Indiana Health Information Exchange (IHIE), Utah Health Information Network (UHIN), and HealthBridge in Cincinnati.

As we mentioned previously, the current era for HIE began in 2004. That was the year that then President George W. Bush signed an Executive Order which established the Office of the National Coordinator for Health Information Technology (ONC) within the U.S. Department of Health & Human Services (HHS). The responsibilities of ONC at its creation were to:

- Provide leadership for the development and implementation of the nationwide health IT infrastructure;
- Advise the Secretary of HHS on health information technology (IT) policies and initiatives; and
- Coordinate the efforts of HHS to meet the goal of making an electronic medical record available for most Americans by 2014.

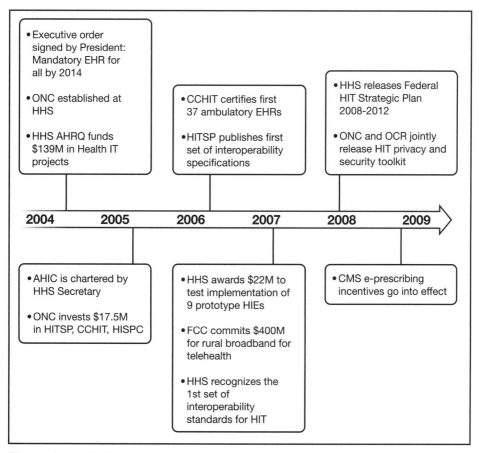

Figure 1-1: HIE Background 2004–2009. © 2009 Mosaica Partners, LLC. Used by permission.

Since its inception, the ONC, along with AHRQ which is also part of HHS, has launched a series of initiatives. The important work from these initiatives has had a significant impact on the HIE landscape of today; thus, we believe that it is crucial that you are aware of these key projects. Figure 1-1 provides a high-level timeline of key federal health information technology initiatives. In the following section, we describe those initiatives in more detail.

Nationwide Health Information Network (NHIN)

A long-term goal of HHS and ONC is to develop a nationwide health information network (NHIN).[2] The NHIN will enable patients, physicians, hospitals, community health centers, public health agencies, laboratories, imaging centers, and other healthcare entities to share clinical information in a secure environment.

In 2004, Phase 1 of the NHIN initiative was launched. This phase consisted of four consortia being tasked to design and evaluate standards-based prototype architectures for the NHIN. Building upon the work done in Phase 1 (the Prototype Architectures), HHS launched Phase 2 (Trial Implementations)[3] in 2007. HHS awarded contracts to nine HIEs to begin trial implementations of the NHIN. Later, an additional six grants were awarded.

This consortium of information exchanges, including providers and several federal agencies, worked together as the *NHIN Cooperative* to securely exchange data, which included summary patient records for providers and patients. In addition to the actual exchange of data, these projects also developed a robust toolset to help in the development and implementation of the NHIN.

Today, in late 2010, the NHIN is operating as the *NHIN Limited Production Exchange*. This network connects a diverse set of federal agencies and private organizations that need to securely exchange electronic health information. These entities currently include the Social Security Administration, MedVirginia, the Department of Veterans Affairs, the Department of Defense, and Kaiser Permanente, among others.

The *NHIN Work Group* (a new workgroup under the HIT Policy Committee—discussed later) was formed to offer recommendations regarding a policy and technical framework that enables the Internet to be used for the secure and standards-based exchange of health information in a way that both fosters innovation and is open to all. At a very high level, the new NHIN Work Group is holding discussions on how to use the Internet to transform healthcare.

After receiving an initial set of recommendations from the NHIN Work Group and others, ONC initiated a new project in the spring of 2010, *NHIN Direct*,[4] to assess and test a working set of specifications to support local health information exchange between providers. As part of this project, a community of stakeholders will collaborate through an open and transparent process to evaluate a set of policies, standards, and services that could enable simple, direct transport of information over the Internet (between providers who know each other). The group will initially focus on the use cases that support meaningful use requirements for 2011. This project is limited in scope with defined outcomes.

Healthcare Information Security and Privacy Collaboration (HISPC)

To address the many conflicting security and privacy regulations, the Healthcare Information Security and Privacy Collaboration Project[5] (HISPC), co-managed by AHRQ and ONC, was launched in 2006. The initial charge to the HISPC project was to enhance the privacy of health information by addressing variations in policies and state laws affecting privacy and security practices. The HISPC project involved more than 40 states and U.S. territories.

The work of Phase 1 of the project focused on the business policies and practices in general, and the security policies and practices in particular, that might hinder the development of effective national, regional, and local systems for electronic health information exchange.

Subsequent phases of the project produced an impact analyses of various state privacy laws affecting HIE. The work in these subsequent phases focused on analyzing consent data elements in state law; studying intrastate and interstate consent policies; developing tools to help harmonize state privacy laws; developing tools and strategies to educate and engage consumers; developing a toolkit to educate providers; recommending basic security policy requirements; and developing model interorganizational agreements.

Health Information Technology Standards Panel (HITSP)

In October, 2005, HHS awarded a $3.3 million contract to the American National Standards Institute (ANSI) to convene the Health Information Technology Standards Panel (HITSP).[6] HITSP is a multidisciplinary coordinating body charged with identifying the technical standards necessary to enable electronic healthcare data interoperability. As of the writing of this book, the contract for HITSP has sunset.

HHS's charge to HITSP was to develop, prototype, and evaluate a harmonization process for achieving a widely accepted and useful set of health IT standards that would support interoperability among healthcare software applications, particularly electronic health records (EHRs). This group was instrumental in identifying and harmonizing standards for health IT. Without the development of these standards, the effective sharing of health information would have remained a nearly insurmountable task.

Certification Commission for Healthcare Information Technology (CCHIT)

The Certification Commission for Health Information Technology (CCHIT)[7] is a private, non-profit organization. Its mission has focused on development of a certification process to accelerate the adoption of health IT by creating an efficient, credible, and sustainable certification program for EHRs. There are more than 200 EHR products on the market today, but until CCHIT was formed in 2006, there were no standard criteria for objectively evaluating their capabilities for sharing data and being interoperable. In 2010, ONC issued the final rule to establish the temporary certification program for EHRs. As of this writing, CCHIT has applied to become an ONC Authorized Testing and Certification Body (ONC-ATCB).

American Health Information Community (AHIC)

The American Health Information Community (AHIC)[8] was a federal advisory body chartered to make recommendations to the Secretary of HHS on how to accelerate the development and adoption of health IT. Prior to the formation of AHIC, there were no agreed-upon standards in place to enable electronic sharing of health information.

From its inauguration in 2005 through November, 2008, AHIC advanced more than 200 recommendations over the course of 25 meetings either in Washington, DC, or at other locations. The recommendations typically addressed a wide variety of enablers and barriers to HIE, such as:
- Standards and certification—for priority areas, which were presented as "use cases";
- Business case—includes public and private sector reimbursement policy;
- Business processes—necessary to integrate health IT into healthcare or consumer management of health;
- Social and cultural issues—includes public awareness and consumer engagement;
- Privacy and security—includes a long list of complex inter-related issues (addressed in detail in Chapter 7, *Protecting Patient Privacy* and Chapter 8, *The Time for Technology*);

- Medical-legal issues—includes liability and licensure of clinicians; and
- The AHIC recommendations to the HHS focused on both consumer/patient needs and population health needs, as well as on the technology/interoperability necessary to advance the use of health information technology (health IT or HIT).

AHIC successfully concluded its operations at the final meeting on November 12, 2008. According to the Secretary's original intent, AHIC was transitioned from a federal advisory committee to a new private-public organization, the National eHealth Collaborative (NeHC).[9] The NeHC intends to work cooperatively and aggressively to accelerate progress on a number of initiatives critical to the achievement of a secure, nationwide electronic health information network.

THE AMERICAN RECOVERY AND REINVESTMENT ACT (ARRA)

And then, along came ARRA—the American Recovery and Reinvestment Act of 2009.

On February 17, 2009, President Barack Obama signed ARRA into law. What ARRA addresses goes far and beyond HIE, but those areas that do address HIE are truly game-changing.

By now, you have heard of the Health Information Technology for Economic and Clinical Health Act (HITECH). This is the section of ARRA that directly addresses health IT. Another section of ARRA addresses the Centers for Medicare & Medicaid Services (CMS) and specifically lays out the requirements and incentives for the Meaningful Use of EHRs. These two sections of the law are the primary federal influences affecting the HIE landscape today. Their impact is, and will continue to be, enormous.

The following is a summary and brief discussion of the health IT-related provisions included in ARRA. Sections of the summary are excerpted from the HIMSS Summary published in July, 2009.[10]

Formal HIE Leadership at the Federal Level

The HITECH Act established formal health IT leadership at the federal level through statute.

Office of the National Coordinator

HITECH established the Office of the National Coordinator for HIT[11] (ONC) and declared that it be headed by a National Coordinator appointed by the Secretary of HHS. The ONC is at the forefront of the federal government's health IT efforts and is a resource to the entire health system to support the adoption of health IT and the promotion of nationwide health information exchange to improve healthcare. ONC is organizationally located within the Office of the Secretary, HHS.

ONC is the federal entity charged with coordination of nationwide efforts to implement and use the most advanced health IT and the electronic exchange of health information. ARRA put the office, formerly established and authorized by executive order, into statute and established the office by federal law. The legislation authorizes and appropriates $2 billion over four years (2009-2012) to fund the ONC.

HIT Policy Committee

The Health IT Policy Committee[12] is charged with making recommendations to the National Coordinator for Health IT on a policy framework to be used for the development and adoption of a nationwide health information infrastructure, including appropriate standards, for the exchange of patient medical information.

HIT Standards Committee

The Health IT Standards Committee[13] is charged with making recommendations to the National Coordinator for Health IT on standards, implementation specifications, and certification criteria for the electronic exchange and use of health information.

Strengthening Privacy and Security Requirements

The HITECH Act specifically addressed privacy and security in several areas.

Security Breach Notification

Under the legislation, a federal security breach notification requirement was established for health information that is not encrypted or otherwise made indecipherable. It requires that individuals be notified if there is an unauthorized disclosure or use of their health information.

New HIPAA Business Associates' Requirements

ARRA strengthens the Health Insurance Portability and Accountability Act (HIPAA) and now ensures that new entities that were not contemplated when HIPAA was written (such as personal health record vendors, RHIOs, HIEs, etc.) are subject to the same privacy and security rules as covered entities (e.g., providers and health insurers), by treating these entities as Business Associates under HIPAA. Because of that change, the HIE organization is now subject to the same privacy and security regulations as covered entities under HIPAA. This is discussed in more detail in Chapter 7, *Protecting Patient Privacy*.

Accounting of Disclosures

ARRA states that patients have the right to request an accounting of any disclosures of their health information that were made through the use of an electronic record.

Sales/Marketing of Protected Health Information (PHI)

ARRA contains new restrictions for using personal health information (PHI) for marketing. It also addresses the circumstances under which an entity can receive remuneration for PHI.

In July, 2010, new proposed regulations under HIPAA were announced by HHS that would restrict disclosures of certain PHI, extend some of the Privacy and Security Rules requirements, expand individuals' rights to access their information, and establish new limitations on the use and disclosure of PHI for marketing and fundraising purposes.[14]

Federal Funding of HIE

Many sources of funding are addressed in ARRA. We will cover three sources that directly relate to your HIE efforts: Meaningful Use Incentives through CMS, Health Information Technology Extension Program, and State Health Information Exchange Cooperative Agreement Program.

Meaningful Use Incentives

ARRA includes billions of dollars in Medicare and Medicaid incentive payments to providers and hospitals to promote the "Meaningful Use" of certified health IT products. These incentives are thoroughly described in the document entitled *Medicare and Medicaid for the Meaningful Use of Certified EHR Technology: Incentive Payments through Medicare and Medicaid for the Meaningful Use of Certified EHR Technology by Eligible Professionals and Hospitals.*[15] The Congressional Budget Office estimates the total cost of providing Medicare and Medicaid incentives for eligible professionals and hospitals that demonstrate a meaningful use of certified EHR technology will be $20.8 billion through fiscal year 2019.

On July 16, 2010, CMS issued the final rule for the Medicare EHR Incentive Program and the Medicaid EHR Incentive program. Detailed information on these programs can be found at the "Official Web Site for the Medicare and Medicaid EHR Incentive Programs."[16]

The Purpose of the Meaningful Use Incentives Law

Congress designed the Meaningful Use legislation[17] to improve U.S. healthcare through the development of a solid electronic health information infrastructure, while simultaneously stimulating the economy through new investment and job growth. The five broad goals for this program are summarized in Figure 1-2.

Incentive Payments to Eligible Providers

An eligible provider will receive incentive payments as specified in the legislation for the first five years (2010–2015), for demonstrating a meaningful use of EHR technology and demonstrating performance during the reporting period for each payment year. To promote rapid adoption of EHR technology, if an eligible professional does not demonstrate meaningful use by 2015, his/her reimbursement payments under Medicare will begin to be reduced. No incentive payment will be made after 2016. Table 1-1 shows an example of the potential reimbursement to eligible Medicare physicians who dem-

---

- Improve quality, safety, efficiency, and reduce health disparities.
- Engage patients and families.
- Improve care coordination.
- Ensure adequate privacy and security protections for personal health information.
- Improve population and public health.

Figure 1-2: Goals of the Meaningful Use Program

Meaningful Use Incentives* by Adoption Year (Physicians)

Meaningful User	2009	2010	2011	2012	2013	2014	2015	2016	Total Incentive
2011			$18,000	$12,000	$ 8,000	$ 4,000	$ 2,000		$44,000
2012				$18,000	$12,000	$ 8,000	$ 4,000	$ 2,000	$44,000
2013					$15,000	$12,000	$ 8,000	$ 4,000	$39,000
2014						$12,000	$ 8,000	$ 4,000	$24,000
2015+									$ Penalties

* Medicare Example

Adapted from the 111th Congress of the United States.
Public Law 111-5—American Recovery and Reinvestment Act of 2009.

Table 1-1: Meaningful Use Incentives for Eligible Medicare Physicians by Adopted Year[18]

onstrate that they are meaningfully using EHRs. The incentives for eligible providers under Medicaid differ somewhat from those for providers under Medicare. They will be administered by each state's Medicaid office.

Progression of Meaningful Use

"Meaningful use of certified EHR technologies" is a term used in the ARRA. It is defined by CMS in a Notice of Proposed Rulemaking (NPRM) as the use of health IT to further the five broad goals of the ARRA and to further the goal of information exchange among health professionals.[19] There is also an Interim Final Rule (IFR) on the Initial Set of Standards, Implementation Specifications, and Certification Criteria for Electronic Health Record Technology.[20] This IFR specifies the standards that an EHR must meet if it is to be certified for the meaningful use criteria. As of this writing, both of these rules have yet to be finalized.

Figure 1-3 shows the progression of the goals that are meant to be achieved through meaningful use:

- Stage 1 efforts are focused on improving the electronic capture and sharing of health information.
- Building on that foundation, stage 2 will focus on implementing advanced clinical practices as we shift from memory-based medicine to information-driven care.
- Stage 3 will focus on showing improved outcomes in the population as healthcare broadly adopts the 21st-century tools available to deliver better treatment outcomes and enhanced disease prevention.

Health Information Technology Regional Extension Program

The HITECH Act authorizes a Health Information Technology Regional Extension Program.[22] The extension program is modeled after the agriculture extension pro-

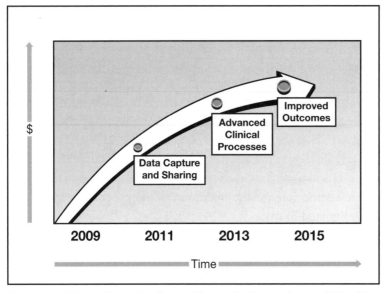

Figure 1-3: Bending the Curve Towards Transformed Healthcare.[21]
Adapted from the Markle Foundation. Achieving the Health IT Objectives of the
American Recovery and Reinvestment Act. *Connecting for Health.* April, 2009.

grams and consists of the establishment of Health IT Regional Extension Centers and a
national Health Information Technology Research Center (HITRC).

Each of the Regional Extension Centers will offer assistance, defined as education,
outreach, and technical assistance, to eligible providers as defined in the ARRA legislation. The objective is to help these healthcare providers located in their geographic
service areas select, successfully implement, and meaningfully use certified EHR technology. This is to be done to support and accelerate healthcare providers' ability to
become meaningful users of EHRs. The programs' objectives are to ensure that primary
care clinicians who need help are provided with an array of on-the-ground support to
meaningfully use EHRs. The specific goal of the program is to provide outreach and
support services to at least 100,000 priority primary care providers nationally within
the first two years.

The HITRC is responsible for gathering relevant information on effective practices
and helping the Regional Extension Centers collaborate with each other and with their
relevant stakeholders. The goal is to identify and share best practices in EHR adoption,
effective use, and provider support.

The federal government has awarded $642,790,024 to 60 organizations to establish
Regional Extension Centers.

State Health Information Exchange Cooperative Agreement Program

Achieving meaningful use of EHRs requires that HIE capability must be present and
available to providers. Recognizing that most states do not currently have this capability in place and widely available, the HITECH Act authorizes the establishment of the
State Health Information Exchange Cooperative Agreement Program.[23] The objective
of this program is to advance appropriate and secure HIE across the healthcare system.
This program funds individual states' efforts to rapidly build capability and capacity for

exchanging health information across the healthcare system—both within and across states. States receiving the awards are responsible for (1) increasing connectivity, and (2) enabling patient-centric information flow to help improve the quality and efficiency of care. Key to this anticipated improvement is the continual evolution and advancement of necessary governance, policies, technical services, business operations, and financing mechanisms for HIE.

The purpose of this program is to continuously improve and expand HIE services to reach all healthcare providers to improve the quality and efficiency of healthcare. The governors of the individual states have the option to designate a state-government or non-government entity to operate the program in their state. Because of this option, the organization in a state responsible for the operation of the program is frequently referred to as the State Designated Entity.

The federal government has awarded $547,703,438 to states and U.S. territories under the State Information Exchange Cooperative Agreement Program.

General Requirements for the First Two Years of the Grant

According to the Request for Grant for funding for the State Health Information Exchange Cooperative Agreement Program,[24] the first two years of the program are critical for building HIE capability. States and their State Designated Entities are expected to make considerable progress in achieving a critical mass of providers participating in HIE during that time. Thus, the majority of the funding available for drawdown will be available in the first two years.

While a state or a State Designated Entity may or may not be the entity to actually implement and operate the technical services to support HIE, they are required to act as the governance entity responsible for ensuring that HIE capability within the state will be developed with appropriate oversight and accountability. The state or State Designated Entity must develop and implement a plan that provides reasonable assurance that the HIE requirements for meaningful use will be attained by 2015—the same year that Medicare penalties begin for providers that have not achieved meaningful use of EHRs.

The following sections show the key requirements the states must meet in the first two years of the four-year grant. The work is divided into five government-defined domains:
- Governance
- Finance
- Technical Infrastructure
- Business and Technical Operations
- Legal/Policy

If you are not familiar with the term "domain," you can think of it as a way to categorize work or activity, typically over time.

Specific Requirements in the Governance Domain

Within the first two years of the grant, states are required to complete the following activities in the Governance domain:

- Establish a governance structure that achieves broad-based stakeholder collaboration with transparency, buy-in, and trust.
- Set goals, objectives and performance measures for the exchange of health information that reflect consensus among the healthcare stakeholder groups and that accomplish statewide coverage of all providers for HIE requirements related to meaningful use criteria.
- Ensure the coordination, integration, and alignment of efforts with Medicaid and public health programs through efforts of the State Health IT Coordinators.
- Establish mechanisms to provide oversight and accountability of HIE to protect the public interest.
- Account for the flexibility needed to align with emerging nationwide HIE governance that will be specified in future program guidance.

Specific Requirements in the Financial Domain

Within the first two years of the grant, states are required to complete the following activities in the Finance domain:

- Develop the capability to effectively manage the funding necessary to implement the state strategic plan.
- Develop a path to sustainability including a business plan with feasible public/private financing mechanisms:
  - For ongoing information exchange among healthcare providers; and
  - With those offering services for patient engagement and information access.

Specific Requirements in the Technical Infrastructure Domain

Within the first two years of the grant, states are required to complete the following activities in the Technical Infrastructure domain:

- Develop, or facilitate the creation of, a statewide technical infrastructure that supports statewide HIE. While states may prioritize among these HIE services according to its needs, the HIE services that must be developed include:
  - Electronic eligibility and claims transactions;
  - Electronic prescribing and refill requests;
  - Electronic clinical laboratory ordering and results delivery;
  - Electronic public health reporting (i.e., immunizations, notifiable laboratory results);
  - Quality reporting;
  - Prescription fill status and/or medication fill history; and
  - Clinical summary exchange for care coordination and patient engagement.
- Leverage any existing regional and state level efforts and resources that can advance HIE, such as master patient indexes, health information organizations (HIOs), and the state's Medicaid Management Information System (MMIS).
- Develop or facilitate the creation and use of shared directories and technical services, as applicable for the state's approach for statewide HIE. Directories may include but are not limited to health care providers, laboratory service providers, radiology service providers, and health plans. Shared services may

include but are not limited to patient matching, provider authentication, consent management, secure routing, advance directives, and messaging.

Specific Requirements in the Business and Technical Operations Domain

Within the first two years of the grant, states are required to complete the following activities in the Business and Technical Operations domain:

- Provide technical assistance as needed to HIEs and others who are developing HIE capacity within the state.
- Coordinate and align efforts to meet Medicaid and public health requirements for HIE and the evolving Meaningful Use criteria.
- Monitor and plan for remediation of the performance of HIE throughout the state.
- Document how the different HIE efforts within the state are enabling meaningful use.

Specific Requirements in the Legal/Policy Domain

Within the first two years of the grant, states are required to complete the following activities in the Legal/Policy domain:

- Identify and harmonize the federal and state legal and policy requirements in order to enable appropriate health information exchange services that are developed in the first two years.
- Establish a statewide policy framework that allows incremental development of HIE policies over time, enables appropriate inter-organizational health information exchange, and meets other important state policy requirements such as those related to public health and vulnerable populations.
- Develop and implement enforcement mechanisms that ensure those implementing and maintaining health information exchange services have appropriate safeguards in place and adhere to legal and policy requirements that protect health information.
- Minimize obstacles in data sharing agreements.
- Ensure that the policies and legal agreements needed to guide the technical services that have been prioritized by the state or State Designated Entity are implemented and then evaluated annually.

Other HITECH Funding Programs

The three programs just described are the broad nationwide programs funded by HHS. HHS is also funding additional targeted programs to promote heath IT and HIE.

Beacon Community Program

In May, 2010, ONC awarded $220 million to 15 Beacon Communities[25] across the U.S. These Beacon Communities will each use the funds to create model programs in their geographical area to demonstrate the benefits of widespread adoption of health IT and HIE to improve the delivery of care for all Americans. They will each generate and disseminate evidence and insights that are applicable to the rest of the nation about the use of health IT resources. The objective is to inform a range of specific clinical, care delivery, and other reforms that, together, can enable the selected communities to achieve measurable and sustainable improvements in healthcare cost, quality, and population health. As of this writing, ONC announced funding opportunities for two additional Beacon Communities, raising the total to 17.

Strategic Health IT Advanced Research Projects (SHARP) Program

The purpose of Strategic Health IT Advanced Research Projects[26] (SHARP) Program awards is to fund research focused on achieving breakthrough advances to address well-documented problems that have, up until now, impeded adoption of health IT: (1) Security of Health Information Technology; (2) Patient-Centered Cognitive Support; (3) Healthcare Application and Network Platform Architectures; and (4) Secondary Use of EHR Data. To date, $60 million has been awarded to four universities.

IT Workforce Development Programs

There are also funds being awarded for IT workforce development.

Curriculum Development Centers[27]—This program provides $10 million in grants to five domestic institutions of higher education to support health IT curriculum development.

Community College Consortia to Educate Health Information Technology Professionals[28]—This program seeks to rapidly create health IT education and training programs at community colleges or expand existing programs. Community colleges funded under this initiative will establish intensive, non-degree training programs that can be completed in six months or less. The consortium is comprised of five regional groups with more than 70 member community colleges in all 50 states that have received grants of $36 million.

Program of Assistance for University-Based Training[29]—The purpose of this program, which has provided $10 million in grants, is to rapidly increase the availability of individuals qualified to serve in specific health IT professional roles that require university-level training.

Competency Examination for Individuals Completing Non-Degree Training[30]—This program provides a $6 million grant to Northern Virginia Community College to support the development and initial administration of a set of health IT competency examinations.

Expanded Access to Broadband

ARRA appropriated $7.2 billion to expand access to broadband services in the U.S. The funding is administered by two federal agencies: (1) the Commerce Department's National Telecommunications and Information Administration (NTIA), which will receive $4.7 billion to administer the *Broadband Technology Opportunities Program*[31];

and (2) the Agriculture Department's Rural Utilities Service, which will receive $2.5 billion to administer the *Broadband Initiatives Program.*

The Broadband Technology Opportunities Program (1) supports the deployment of broadband infrastructure; (2) enhances and expands public computer centers, such as those found in public libraries; (3) encourages sustainable adoption of broadband service; and (4) develops and maintains a nationwide public map of broadband service capability and availability.

The Broadband Initiatives Program will furnish loans, grants, and loan/grant combinations to assist with addressing the challenge of rapidly expanding the access and quality of broadband services across rural America.

Technical Standards and Certification

ARRA specified that ONC should issue standards and certification criteria for the certification of EHR technology. On July 28, 2010, ONC published the Standards and Certification Criteria Final Rule in the *Federal Register.* This rule describes the requirements that EHRs must meet to ensure they offer the "necessary technological capability, functionality, and security to help them meet the Meaningful Use criteria established for a given phase."[32]

To address the immediate needs for EHR certification for meaningful use, ONC initiated a temporary certification program to certify that EHRs are capable of assisting providers to meet the Meaningful Use criteria. Applications to become an ONC-Authorized Testing and Certification Body (ONC-ATCB) were being accepted as of the writing of this book (summer 2010).

THE HITECH VISION

All of the organizations and programs previously mentioned have been initiated to improve the quality of healthcare. The provisions of the HITECH Act are specifically designed to work together to:

- Provide the necessary assistance and technical support to providers to assist them to achieve Meaningful Use of EHRs;
- Enable coordination and alignment of HIE efforts and resources within and among states;
- Establish connectivity to the public health community in case of emergencies; and
- Ensure the workforce is properly trained and equipped to be meaningful users of EHRs.

Figure 1-4 provides a high-level summary of how the programs are envisioned to work together.

The **OBJECTIVE** is improved healthcare and improved patient outcomes through the use of EHRs and the sharing of health information.

The **Regional Extension Centers** provide direct support to providers in helping them meet the requirements of using EHRs to meet the Meaningful Use criteria and improve care.

The **State Designated Entities** and **HIEs** provide the infrastructure— legal, governance, services and technology—to enable the providers to exchange health information in order to reach the objective of improved quality of care.

Workforce training programs provide trained personnel in the area of IT.

Broadband programs provide the basic Internet connectivity— especially in rural areas that have traditionally been underserved in their communications capability.

Figure 1-4: State HIE Collaborative and HIT Extension Center Program Support

The provisions of the HITECH Act are best understood *not as investments in technology*, but as *efforts to improve the health of Americans and the performance of the healthcare system.* According to Dr. David Blumenthal, the current National Coordinator for HIT, "HITECH Act programs and regulations address the most pressing obstacles to the adoption and meaningful use of EHRs and strive to create an electronic circulatory system for health information that nourishes the practice of medicine, research, and public health, making health care professionals better at what they do and the American people healthier." Figure 1-5 shows the concept of how the various programs within ONC are envisioned to support each other and the objective of improved patient outcomes.

As described previously, the State HIE Cooperative Agreement Programs and the HIT Regional Extension Center programs are being put into place as resources to help you as you form and operate your HIE. It is critical that you also become familiar with the programs created in your own state. Get to know the people involved with these programs. Consider actively involving them in your planning and formation efforts. It is important that you take advantage of all the resources available to you.

Now that you are equipped with a high-level understanding of the environment in which you will be forming your HIE, *let's get started!*

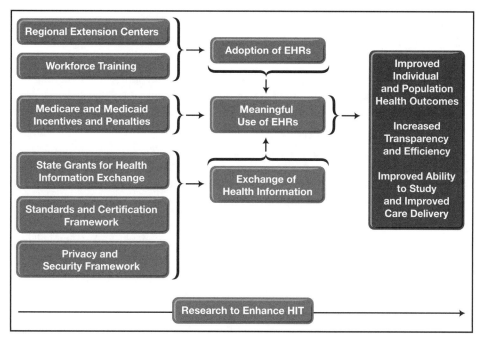

Figure 1-5: The HITECH Vision. Adapted from the Department of Health & Human Services, Office of the National Coordinator for Health Information Technology.[33] Celebrating the First Anniversary of the HITECH Act and Looking to the Future. February, 2010.

REFERENCES

1. HIMSS. *HIMSS Dictionary of Healthcare Information Technology Terms, Acronyms and Organizations, Second Edition.* Chicago: HIMSS; 2010.

2. Department of Health & Human Services, Office of the National Coordinator for Health Information Technology. Nationwide Health Information Network (NHIN): Overview. http://healthit.hhs.gov/portal/server.pt?open=512&objID=1142&parentname=CommunityPage&parentid=16&mode=2&in_hi_userid=10741&cached=true. Accessed April, 2010.

3. Department of Health & Human Services, Office of the National Coordinator for Health Information Technology, Nationwide Health Information Network (NHIN): Trial Implementations. http://healthit.hhs.gov/portal/server.pt?open=512&objID=1191&parentname=CommunityPage&parentid=9&mode=2&in_hi_userid=10732&cached=true. Accessed April, 2010.

4. The NHIN Direct Project. http://nhindirect.org/.

5. Department of Health & Human Services, Office of the National Coordinator for Health Information Technology. The Health Information Privacy and Security Collaboration (HISPC). http://healthit.hhs.gov/portal/server.pt?open=512&mode=2&cached=true&objID=1240. Accessed April, 2010.

6. Healthcare Information Technology Standards Panel (HITSP). Frequently Asked Questions. http://www.hitsp.org/faq.aspx#formed/. Accessed April, 2010.

7. Certification Commission for Health Information Technology (CCHIT). About the Certification Commission for Health Information Technology. http://www.cchit.org/about. Accessed April, 2010.

8. Department of Health & Human Services, Office of the National Coordinator for Health Information Technology. American Health Information Community (AHIC). http://healthit.hhs.gov/portal/server.pt?open=512&mode=2&cached=true&objID=1199. Accessed April, 2010.

9. National eHealth Collaborative. http://www.nationalehealth.org/. Accessed April, 2010.

10. HIMSS. Summary of Key Health Information Technology Provisions, July 1, 2009. http://www.himss. org/content/files/HIMSS_SummaryOfARRA.pdf. Accessed April, 2010.

11. Department of Health & Human Services, Office of the National Coordinator for Health Information Technology. The Office of the National Coordinator for Health Information Technology (ONC). http://healthit.hhs.gov/portal/server.pt?open=512&objID=1200&parentname=CommunityPage& parentid=10&mode=2&in_hi_userid=10741&cached=true. Accessed April, 2010.

12. Department of Health & Human Services, Office of the National Coordinator for Health Information Technology. Health IT Policy Committee (a Federal Advisory Committee). http://healthit.hhs.gov/ portal/server.pt?open=512&objID=1269&parentname=CommunityPage&parentid=4&mode=2&in_ hi_userid=11113&cached=true. Accessed April, 2010.

13. Department of Health & Human Services, Office of the National Coordinator for Health Information Technology. Health IT Standards Committee (a Federal Advisory Committee). http://healthit.hhs. gov/portal/server.pt?open=512&objID=1271&parentname=CommunityPage&parentid=6&mode=2. Accessed April, 2010.

14. Office of the National Coordinator Health Information Technology. Building Trust in Health Information   Exchange.   http://healthit.hhs.gov/portal/server.pt?CommunityID=2994&spaceID=11& parentname=CommunityEditor&control=SetCommunity&parentid=9&in_hi_userid=11673& PageID=0&space=CommunityPage. Accessed August, 2010.

15. Congress of the United States. Public Law 111 - 5 - American Recovery and Reinvestment Act of 2009. http://www.gpo.gov/fdsys/pkg/PLAW-111publ5/content-detail.html. Accessed April, 2010.

16. Centers for Medicare & Medicaid Services, The Official Web Site for the Medicare and Medicaid EHR Incentive Programs. http://www.cms.gov/ehrincentiveprograms/. Accessed August, 2010.

17. HIMSS. The Basics; Frequently Asked Questions on Meaningful Use and the American Recovery and Reinvestment Act of 2009, January 21, 2010. http://www.himss.org/content/files/ BasicFactsAboutMeaningfulUseARRA.pdf. Accessed April, 2010.

18. Adapted from the 111th Congress of the United States. Public Law 111 - 5 - American Recovery and Reinvestment Act of 2009. http://www.gpo.gov/fdsys/pkg/PLAW-111publ5/content-detail.html. Accessed April, 2010.

19. Department of Health & Human Services, Office of the National Coordinator for Health Information Technology. Meaningful Use Notice of Proposed Rulemaking (NPRM). Posted January 13, 2010. http://edocket.access.gpo.gov/2010/E9-31217.htm. Accessed April, 2010.

20. Department of Health & Human Services, Office of the National Coordinator for Health Information Technology. Standards & Certification Criteria IFR. http://healthit.hhs.gov/portal/server. pt?open=512&objID=1195&parentname=CommunityPage&parentid=65&mode=2&in_hi_ userid=11673&cached=true. Accessed April, 2010.

21. Adapted from the Markle Foundation. Achieving the Health IT Objectives of the American Recovery and Reinvestment Act. Connecting for Health. April, 2009. http://www.connectingforhealth.org/arra/ strategic3.html. Accessed April, 2010.

22. Department of Health & Human Services, Office of the National Coordinator for Health Information Technology. Health Information Technology Extension Program. http://healthit.hhs.gov/portal/ server.pt?open=512&objID=1335&mode=2&cached=true. Accessed April, 2010.

23. Department of Health & Human Services, Office of the National Coordinator for Health Information Technology. State Health Information Exchange Cooperative Agreement Program. http://healthit.hhs.

gov/portal/server.pt?open=512&objID=1488&parentname=CommunityPage&parentid=21&mode= 2&in_hi_userid=10741&cached=true. Accessed April, 2010.

24. Department of Health & Human Services, Office of the National Coordinator for Health Information Technology. State Health Information Exchange Cooperative Agreement Program. http://healthit.hhs. gov/portal/server.pt?open=512&objID=1336&parentname=CommunityPage&parentid=10&mode= 2&in_hi_userid=11113&cached=true. Accessed April, 2010.

25. Office of the National Coordinator for Health Information Technology, Beacon Community Program. http://healthit.hhs.gov/portal/server.pt/community/healthit_hhs_gov__beacon_community_pro-gram/1805. Accessed August, 2010.

26. Office of the National Coordinator for Health Information Technology, Strategic Health IT Advanced Research Projects (SHARP) Program. http://healthit.hhs.gov/portal/server.pt?open=512&objID=1 806&parentname=CommunityPage&parentid=17&mode=2&in_hi_userid=11673&cached=true. Accessed August, 2010.

27. Office of the National Coordinator for Health Information Technology. Curriculum Development Centers Program. http://healthit.hhs.gov/portal/server.pt?open=512&objID=1807&parentname= CommunityPage&parentid=13&mode=2&in_hi_userid=11673&cached=true. Accessed August, 2010.

28. Office of the National Coordinator for Health Information Technology, Community College Con-sortia to Educate Health Information Technology Professionals in Health Care Program. http:// healthit.hhs.gov/portal/server.pt?open=512&objID=1804&parentname=CommunityPage&parentid= 14&mode=2&in_hi_userid=11673&cached=true. Accessed August, 2010.

29. Office of the National Coordinator for Health Information Technology, Program of Assistance for University-Based Training. http://healthit.hhs.gov/portal/server.pt?open=512&objID=1808& parentname=CommunityPage&parentid=15&mode=2&in_hi_userid=11673&cached=true. Accessed August, 2010.

30. Office of the National Coordinator for Health Information Technology, Competency Examination for Individuals Completing Non-Degree Training. http://healthit.hhs.gov/portal/server.pt?open= 512&objID=1809&parentname=CommunityPage&parentid=16&mode=2&in_hi_userid=11673& cached=true. Accessed August, 2010.

31. BroadbandUSA. Connecting America's Communities. Broadband Technology Opportunities Pro-gram. http://www2.ntia.doc.gov/about. Accessed August, 2010.

32. Office of the National Coordinator for Health Information Technology. Electronic Health Records and Meaningful Use. http://healthit.hhs.gov/portal/server.pt/community/healthit_hhs_gov_ meaningful_use_announcement/2996. Accessed August, 2010.

33. Adapted from the Department of Health & Human Services, Office of the National Coordinator for Health Information Technology. Celebrating the First Anniversary of the HITECH Act and Looking to the Future. Posted February, 2010. http://healthit.hhs.gov/portal/server.pt?open=18&objID=910780& parentname=CommunityPage&parentid=9&mode=2&in_hi_userid=10741&cached=true. Accessed April, 2010.

CHAPTER 2

Getting Started

The engagement of your stakeholders—and their active and ongoing participation—is the key to your success.

INTRODUCTION

You may be reading this guide because you're interested in forming a health information exchange organization in your state or region. On the other hand, you may be seeking to learn more about what an HIE is and its role in improving healthcare. If you're like most people, you're probably wondering where to start. How do you determine and initiate the activities, and generate the needed participation that will set you on the path to successful and sustainable sharing of secure health information? How do you get started? Where do you begin?

This book, based on our research and hands-on experience in working with states, regions, and communities, is about forming a health information exchange and the various activities that need to be completed for an HIE to become operational. We start with a short discussion of how to begin and then throughout the book provide in-depth discussions and guidance on the journey of forming an HIE. This is your path to a successful, operational HIE.

In this chapter, we help you get started by describing the first steps toward health information exchange. We discuss the things that you need to do to get started—and how to involve your stakeholders early and often. The approach we describe provides a solid foundation upon which to build your successful HIE.

Here, we take you through forming your initial Exploratory Committee and engaging various stakeholder segments from your community and state. Throughout this book, we will remind you repeatedly of how critical it is to continuously identify and engage your various stakeholders. Their needs may change over time, and how you work with them may change, but the fact that you need to keep your stakeholders engaged—and their needs at the forefront of all of your efforts—will never change.

In later chapters, we discuss setting up your governance, developing your business plan, and creating your technical architecture. All of these are important components of your HIE, but no component is more important than consistently involving your key stakeholders all along the way. Without your stakeholders, there will be no need for governance, no possibility of a sustainable business plan, and no need for technology because there will be no participation and no information available to exchange.

While the definition of the term *stakeholder* may vary among HIEs, in this book we use it to refer to anyone who is involved with, affected by, or who influences the sharing of health information. The relative importance and role of different stakeholder groups will vary over time, and your own community characteristics will determine who *your* stakeholders are and how they will be involved.

As Jeff Blair from the NMHIC advises, "Be patient, include anyone that is interested. Community organizing takes a long time. Stakeholders for HIE require community organizing at the executive level."

THE FIVE STAGES OF THE HIE ORGANIZATIONAL LIFECYCLE

Based on our experience, a health information exchange goes through several stages during its lifetime. It starts with an idea. Figure 2-1 summarizes the stages of the HIE lifecycle.

Initiation

The idea for an HIE often starts with just a few people who are passionate about improving the quality of healthcare in their region or community. The idea then spreads to a few more people who are motivated to help. Soon there is an Exploratory Committee that, after further investigation, decides to begin the efforts to form an HIE.

Formation

Once the Exploratory Committee determines that an HIE is the right approach for their community and that there is sufficient interest, the journey of forming an HIE begins in earnest. Forming an HIE is a significant project that consumes a lot of effort and resources. And it takes time. It has been described by some as similar to taking a dozen cats for a walk. Formation takes you through the steps that turn that initial idea for an HIE into a reality. The formation stage is the topic of this book.

Operation

The operation stage begins when an HIE is "open for business" and the exchange is running and live data are actually being exchanged. This is when you begin to see the fruits of all of your labors in the formation stage. The community, and the individuals

---

- Initiation
- Formation
- Operation
- Optimization
- Consolidation

Figure 2-1: HIE Lifecycle Stages

in it, begin to benefit from the availability of more complete patient information at the point of care.

Optimization

Optimization begins when you implement various new services and start to analyze and respond to your performance metrics. During the optimization stage, you fine tune your processes and become more efficient and more effective at providing the information and support necessary to deliver better care and improve health outcomes. Stakeholders are consistently involved as they determine new ways to use the HIE and become more involved in developing additional services. Working with them, you can develop new service offerings as you strive to better meet their needs.

Consolidation

Consolidation is the stage that we believe is yet to come. As the need for more and better patient information, and the results of using more complete data, are woven into the fabric of our healthcare environment, we believe that there will be increased demands for HIE services and capabilities. As we have seen in many other business sectors, these increased demands will cause new thinking about how to leverage economies of scale. Successful HIEs will merge or consolidate to provide more and better services on an increasingly cost-effective basis.

THE FIVE HIE COMPETENCY AND ACTIVITY DOMAINS

We believe that there are five domains that need to be addressed when forming an HIE. These are:

- Stakeholder Engagement & Participation
- Governance
- Business & Finance
- Privacy
- Technology & Security

These domains represent both (1) the categories of activity involved in the building of an HIE, and (2) the specific areas of personal and professional competence needed from the people who assist with, and participate in, the process of forming your HIE.

In this book, we group the domains a bit differently than the domains the federal government identified in its description of the work of the State Designated Entities (see Chapter 1, *The HIE Landscape*). We believe that the efforts to form a regional HIE involve a somewhat different focus from those of developing the statewide capabilities to support health information exchange.

Stakeholder Engagement & Participation

Description: The identification, organization, motivation, coordination, and active communication with various disparate stakeholders throughout the entire process of initiating, forming, operating, optimizing, and consolidating an HIE.

Typical activities involve surveying and assessing the community; identifying stakeholders with an interest in the HIE; developing and executing the communication plan; identifying stakeholders who are candidates for roles in the organization; identifying early funding sources; preparing and delivering presentations; and proactively maintaining ongoing contact with stakeholders.

Personal and professional competences include the ability to do the following: determine, understand, rank and prioritize the wants and needs of the different categories of stakeholders that have been identified; coordinate a group of disparate stakeholders with different wants and needs, and help them arrive at a consensus on issues; clearly communicate the benefits of HIE to the community and the various stakeholder groups within it; develop and execute a communication plan; and most importantly, dialogue with your stakeholders.

Governance

Description: The identification, evaluation, and use of various organizational governance models and approaches to ensure the organization is developing and operating in a reasonable, appropriate, and legal manner.

Typical activities involve establishing the initial committees and organizational frameworks (organizing committee, development committees, board, operating committees, business structure and approach) and developing and monitoring the specific approaches those organizations will use in the setting of principles and policies.

Personal and professional competences include the ability to do the following: establish an organization; evaluate different organizational formation options; provide practical guidance through the entire HIE planning, formation and operations stages; seek out and understand legal guidance relative to the applicable laws and regulations; and view and coordinate the development of the HIE as a significant change management project.

Business & Finance

Description: The evaluation, selection and oversight of appropriate legal entity structures and financial models and approaches for the HIE.

Typical activities involve comparing various business legal structures; developing initial, interim and operating budgets; determining early funding requirements; ensuring the organization is established in conformance with local, regional, and state laws; approving contracts with external parties; and setting up and managing the organization's books and accounts.

Personal and professional competences include the ability to do the following: provide business and financial guidance through the entire HIE process; negotiate contracts for goods and services; evaluate different business models and potential funding sources; set up and monitor accounting systems; and manage and direct the efforts of volunteers and paid staff members to achieve defined objectives.

Privacy

Description: Ensuring the various federal, state, and local laws and regulations related to keeping protected health information private are understood and enforced by the HIE.

Typical activities involve investigating and understanding the differences between federal and state laws and regulations; coordinating with the state's State Designated Entity to ensure a harmonization of efforts related to privacy; developing privacy policies; and providing input to the technical requirements in areas related to privacy.

Personal and professional competences include the ability to do the following: understand and communicate all appropriate statutes and regulations including the latest updates to HIPAA, and clearly communicate the requirements of those statutes and regulations to fellow team members who have responsibility for evaluating and selecting the technology infrastructure that will be used by the HIE.

Technology & Security

Description: The evaluation, creation and implementation of an appropriate technical architecture for the HIE. Understanding of various approaches and technologies used to secure personal health information. Understanding, describing, and differentiating between various technical architecture models and approaches. Providing technical guidance through the entire HIE formation and operations stages.

Typical activities involve researching various technical architecture models based on both business and privacy requirements; developing security policies to complement the privacy policies; evaluating various technology component options; developing testing and validation approaches; coordinating the technical transition from a testing environment to a pilot environment and then to a production environment; and ensuring appropriate audit and control mechanisms are in place to ensure conformance to statutes and regulations.

Personal and professional competences include the ability to evaluate and specify technical infrastructure components to ensure that the HIE is operating in a manner consistent with its business policies and procedures and in compliance with all appropriate statues and regulations; an understanding of the security requirements needed to comply with all relevant federal and state laws and regulations; an understanding of the technical implementation of security policies; a working knowledge of tools used to safeguard security; the ability to manage a complex technical development or implementation project; the ability to define and establish process control and monitoring mechanisms to ensure the technology components are operating according to specification; and the ability to validate that the infrastructure components chosen by the HIE are in conformance with security policies.

Each of these five domains includes specific milestones to be reached, and capabilities to build, in the various phases of an HIE's formation stage. Many of these capabilities are dependent upon activities that cross domains and involve multiple skills. Figure 2-2 illustrates the HIE Maturity Framework we have developed. It shows how our five domains and the five stages of the HIE Lifecycle relate to each other.

As you move through the formation stage, you'll be continuously building upon and enhancing the capabilities that you previously developed. Forming an HIE is not easy, but it is doable. There is a path—with some clearly defined steps—and it is one that others have navigated successfully. You can do it, too. Take one step at a time and just keep heading in the right direction.

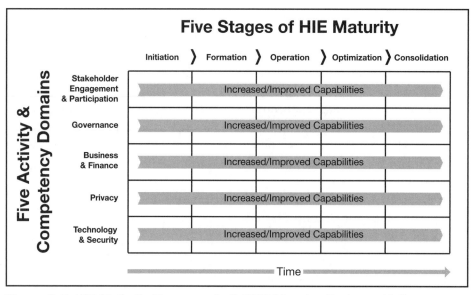

Figure 2-2: HIE Maturity Framework. © 2009 Mosaica Partners, LLC.
Used by permission.

STEPS TO GETTING STARTED

You will start on the path to exchanging health information with the initial step of forming your core team. We will show you where to begin and what objectives you need to achieve as you start your journey toward successful operation. Figure 2-3 summarizes the steps that will help you get started on your HIE formation journey.

INITIATION STAGE

You have an idea. You also have the passion. You know that healthcare can be improved by electronically sharing patient health information. Congratulations. You have entered the Initiation Stage.

Form Your Exploratory Committee

The first thing you need to do is to find others in your community who are interested in, and willing to become part of, the core team necessary to get your efforts moving. Talk to people in your community, and identify those who are willing to commit their time, talent, and resources to assess whether your community is ready for HIE. Look for people who are passionate about making this change a reality. Find people with the right skills and personality to enable them to communicate the idea to others and motivate them to participate. Seek out community leaders—people who are influential in and familiar with your community—who have a passion for improving healthcare.

According to Liesa Jenkins, CareSpark started by identifying individuals who had a passion and interest [in HIE]. She says, "If you can find those and they're willing to commit, they are the missionaries who make converts of others."

The words and phrases we often hear when people describe the types of individuals who should be involved in the Exploratory Committee are "passion," "commitment," "understand it's about the greater good," "able to set aside their own agendas," "believe

---

Initiation
   1. Form your Exploratory Committee.

Formation
   2. Reach out to your community.
   3. Understand your community.
   4. Engage your stakeholders.
   5. Develop your communication plan.
   6. Engage with your State Designated Entity.
   7. Engage with your Regional Extension Center.

Figure 2-3: The Steps for Getting Started

that it needs to be done," and "care about the patient." These descriptive phrases should apply to the people you approach to become members of your team.

It is critical that you involve physicians at the onset. Every community has physicians who believe that better information will make them better healthcare providers. Find them and get them involved early in the project. Michael Matthews of MedVirginia emphasizes the importance of provider engagement by recommending that those forming an HIE "get close to the physicians and gain their trust…Win the hearts and minds of the physicians. If you do that, others will also be interested in participation."

It is important to involve a good cross-section of your community, particularly your healthcare community, even at this early stage. You may find that some of the larger healthcare institutions in your community are reluctant to become involved. Keep looking. You will find someone from a hospital or large provider practice who believes in your cause. If you do not find him or her right away, keep moving forward anyway. That person will join you when the time is right.

At this stage, you may only have a small group of stakeholders involved. That's okay. We'll show you how to expand participation and engage others in your efforts as we move through the following chapters together.

Once you have gathered this initial small core group, hold your first Exploratory Committee meeting. This can be an informal meeting, perhaps over coffee, but be sure to prepare a focused agenda. In Figure 2-4, we provide an example of some of the items to consider when preparing your agenda.

Plan to hold several of these Exploratory Committee meetings. You need to keep involving people until you have enough information and sufficient participation to enable you to move forward.

The Exploratory Committee needs to become familiar with activities surrounding HIE development at the national and state level. The committee also needs to be aware of any related activities in your region. Things are changing rapidly in today's environment, so it is essential that you have at least a high-level understanding of the HIE environment, including the many resources and funding opportunities available. In Chapter 1, *The HIE Landscape*, we provided an overview of today's national HIE landscape. Here we provide some options for additional ways of becoming more informed

1. Discuss what an HIE is and how you can determine if this is the right time for your community.

2. Hold an informal discussion among the participants on their perspectives of the community regarding readiness for HIE.

3. Discuss who else from the community should be invited to join the committee.

4. Identify a note taker and take notes in the meeting. This may be a rather informal meeting, but some notes from the meeting may be helpful as you move forward.

5. Identify other HIE organizations in your state or region to which you may want to reach out.

6. Identify next actions, develop a short list of action items to accomplish before the next meeting, and assign the tasks—such as who else should be involved, who will contact whom, etc.

7. Schedule the next meeting within the following two weeks.

8. Make sure you follow up on the assignments from this meeting.

Figure 2-4: Exploratory Committee Meeting Agenda Items to Consider

about HIE. Figure 2-5 suggests activities for gaining more information on HIEs and their formation.

FORMATION STAGE

Once your Exploratory Committee understands the purpose of HIE and decides there is sufficient interest, need, and support in the community for HIE, you move into the formation stage. You will remain in this stage until you are officially "open for business" and exchanging health information electronically.

The actual process of planning your HIE is critical. Experience shows that while the planning stage should not be too short—less than six months is typically not long enough to complete your planning activities and gain the appropriate level of support—it should not be too long, either. Planning efforts longer than 18 months tend to fatigue the participants, who are primarily volunteers, and can create doubt in the community as they wonder whether this project will ever get off the ground and actually deliver the needed capabilities for health information exchange.

As you continue to explore your community, you begin the activities that move your exploratory group toward an agreement to proceed with building the HIE. In your efforts to achieve this agreement, you undertake specific fact-finding activities relating to your community. This adds to the knowledge and perspectives already contributed by your committee members.

- Bring in someone knowledgeable in the HIE environment for a half-day or full-day briefing.
- Schedule a series of webinars to which you have invited speakers who are directly involved with HIE at the regional, state, or national level.
- Attend other readily available free or low-cost webinars put on by professional or trade organizations, such as HIMSS.
- Review the resource websites listed at the end of Chapter 1, *The HIE Landscape.*
- Initiate communication with your state's State Designated Entity and your state's Health Information Regional Extension Center to understand how their efforts can complement those in your community.

Figure 2-5: Ideas for Educating the Exploratory Committee on HIE

Understand Your Community at a High Level

In our consulting practice, we have found that healthcare, like politics, is local. Each HIE reflects its community's size, culture, and mores. It is now time to conduct an initial high-level assessment of your community. There will be more in-depth information gathering later, but at this stage, you need to gain a basic understanding of your environment from a healthcare provider perspective. This is necessary so that you understand the environment in which you will form and operate your HIE.

The more information you can gather about your community, the better your understanding will be. Examples of the kind of information you should gather include:

- How many hospitals are there, and what are their sizes?
- How many physicians and other key health providers are practicing, and what is the mix of specialties?
- How many and what kind of ancillary service providers—such as labs, radiology, and pharmacies—are in your area?
- How many and what types of community health centers, long-term care facilities and assisted living communities are in your area?
- Who are the key people at the organizations you want to involve?
- What are the demographics of your community—age, ethnic make up, language, stable or transient population, and prevalent languages?
- Who are the people with influence in your community?
- Who are the major stakeholder groups in your community, especially those with a clear stake in healthcare?
- What are the external factors that will impact your formation?

In later chapters, we discuss how you can gain a more in-depth understanding of the specific needs your community will want the HIE to meet, but at this point, you only need to gain a basic understanding of the community as a whole. However, this initial community assessment is critical for you. You will use it over and over as you engage stakeholders and work to sustain their interest through the various stages of

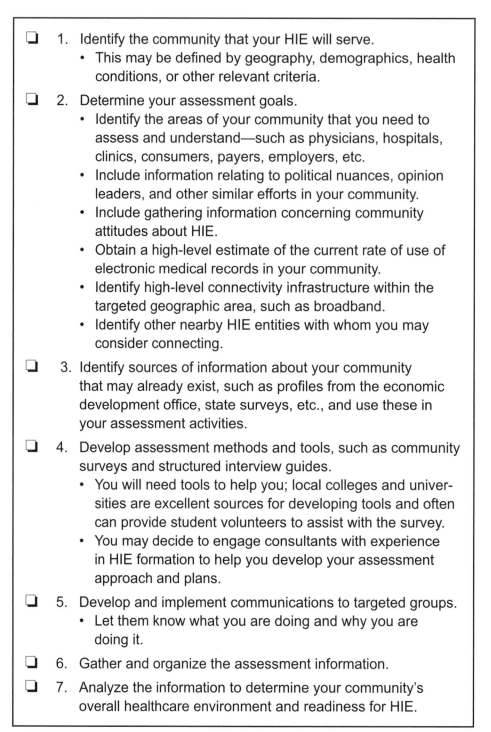

❏   1. Identify the community that your HIE will serve.
        • This may be defined by geography, demographics, health
          conditions, or other relevant criteria.

❏   2. Determine your assessment goals.
        • Identify the areas of your community that you need to
          assess and understand—such as physicians, hospitals,
          clinics, consumers, payers, employers, etc.
        • Include information relating to political nuances, opinion
          leaders, and other similar efforts in your community.
        • Include gathering information concerning community
          attitudes about HIE.
        • Obtain a high-level estimate of the current rate of use of
          electronic medical records in your community.
        • Identify high-level connectivity infrastructure within the
          targeted geographic area, such as broadband.
        • Identify other nearby HIE entities with whom you may
          consider connecting.

❏   3. Identify sources of information about your community
        that may already exist, such as profiles from the economic
        development office, state surveys, etc., and use these in
        your assessment activities.

❏   4. Develop assessment methods and tools, such as community
        surveys and structured interview guides.
        • You will need tools to help you; local colleges and univer-
          sities are excellent sources for developing tools and often
          can provide student volunteers to assist with the survey.
        • You may decide to engage consultants with experience
          in HIE formation to help you develop your assessment
          approach and plans.

❏   5. Develop and implement communications to targeted groups.
        • Let them know what you are doing and why you are
          doing it.

❏   6. Gather and organize the assessment information.

❏   7. Analyze the information to determine your community's
        overall healthcare environment and readiness for HIE.

Figure 2-6: Checklist—Initial Assessment of Community

HIE formation and operation. Use the checklist in Figure 2-6 as a guide to help you
determine your approach to your initial community assessment.

Additional things you need to be on the lookout for as you assess your community
are barriers that may prevent you from being successful, such as reluctance on the part

of some providers to share data; their concerns about costs; or their questions about protecting patient privacy. Document these barriers. You will use this information to make sure you address the barriers as you build your plan. At the same time, identify community priorities that you can leverage to propel your efforts forward.

For example, there are many times when natural disasters, such as hurricanes or floods, have propelled a community's efforts to establish an HIE. There may be other factors in your community, such as a high prevalence of chronic disease or other risk factors, that provide leverage for implementing HIE as a means to improving healthcare. Use this information to determine where the pain points exist in your community.

There are almost as many reasons for starting an HIE as there are HIEs in operation.

For example, the reason for initiating CareSpark, which serves rural areas in Tennessee, Virginia, and Kentucky, was grounded in the recognition that the community had poor health status and needed to work together to improve that status. Their mission focuses on the total community with the underlying thought, according to Liesa Jenkins, that "if you're going to change community health, you need everybody there—public health, media, healthcare, consumers, everybody—to help change that."

On the other hand, HealthBridge can trace its beginnings to an unsuccessful CHIN effort in the 1990s. At that time, the major employers in the region were very interested in using technology to improve the quality and economics of healthcare in their region. One approach they considered was centralizing pay claims information. While the providers were not generally in favor of this approach, the overall threat of this happening outside of their control solidified the provider community to work together.

As you assess your community, it is important to determine if there is enough interest in HIE and if there are a sufficient number and type of key stakeholders who will support your efforts. In addition to understanding your community's interest and readiness for HIE, you need to take the "technical temperature" of the community. This will provide you with a high-level estimate of the current level of EHR adoption and the health IT priorities in your community. The national average for physician adoption of full EHRs is less than 20%. How does your community compare?

It's okay if you discover that there is a lot of preparatory work that needs to be completed in your community before you can exchange health information. That's typical, and it's the reason for the formation stage. There are few, if any, communities today that are fully prepared for HIE.

THE IMPORTANCE OF BEGINNING WITH STAKEHOLDER ENGAGEMENT AND PARTICIPATION

Stakeholder engagement and participation is key to your HIE success. This requires you to establish and maintain the interest, commitment, and participation of various groups of stakeholders throughout the entire life cycle of the HIE. The goal of stakeholder sustainability must permeate the entire organization and its processes.

Now is the time to build the foundation of a sustainable HIE. Simply stated, your success depends on your stakeholders and how you treat them. If you involve them early, get them engaged, and keep them involved and participating, they will be more likely to participate in the HIE as it becomes operational. If you fail to successfully

---

Identify your key stakeholders.
  - How do you know if you have the right types of stakeholders?
  - How do you find them?
  - How do you engage them?
  - How do you keep them?

Get commitment from your key stakeholders.
  - If you cannot get their commitment, either you are not
    designing the right kind of HIE or you have not involved
    the right stakeholders.

Figure 2-7: Identifying and Engaging the Right Stakeholders

engage your stakeholders at the beginning and throughout your formation efforts, you will have no choice but to go back to the beginning and try to engage them again—and that is not easy to do.

In Chapter 4, *Establish a Formal Organizational Governance Structure*, we discuss the stakeholder engagement workgroup that you will create to lead stakeholder engagement efforts during the formation of your HIE. In this chapter, we discuss the background and early activities that relate to the work of this group. Refer back to this chapter when you are ready to launch your stakeholder engagement workgroup.

In our experience, we have encountered many failed and failing HIE efforts that began with the belief, "If you build it, they will come." This is a dangerous misconception, and it will hurt your efforts. You can build it, but if your stakeholders are not involved all along the way, they will not be there when you want them to participate. Figure 2-7 lists areas to consider as you develop your stakeholder engagement plans.

We also have seen efforts which started with a large group of interested stakeholders, but failed in their efforts to form an HIE because their leadership team did not pay attention to their stakeholders at every step along the way. Conversely, the leaders of every successful HIE that we have worked with, or interviewed for this book, could not emphasize strongly enough the importance of communicating with stakeholders and keeping them involved at every step.

Your community assessment will identify some of the individuals who are opinion leaders in your state or your community and who also believe in the promise of HIE. These people are typically enthusiastic about improving patient care by electronically sharing health information. Nurture them. Encourage them. Involve them early in your planning efforts. If you build your HIE with their active involvement, chances are very good that they will be among the first to participate when you are operational.

Consider the characteristics of your community and the various types of stakeholder groups it contains. To help you think through and identify the various types of stakeholder groups in your community, we provide a broad list of potential stakeholders in Figure 2-8 for you to consider.

Regardless of whether you are forming a state or regional HIE, you need strong stakeholder involvement. As we have stated, our experience clearly shows how important stakeholder engagement is—from the very earliest stage of the HIE. Throughout

Stakeholder groups that you may want to include:
- Behavioral Health Centers
- Community Colleges
- Community Health Centers and Rural Health Clinics
- Consumer and Patient Groups
- Department of Health (State, County and City)
- Economic Development Organizations
- Emergency Medical Services Providers
- Employers (especially large employers)
- Government – Federal, State, and Local
- Health Center Controlled Networks (HCCNs)
- Health Plans and Payers
- Health Professional Societies
- Hospitals and Hospital Systems
- Laboratories
- Long-term Care Providers
- Medical Societies
- Medicare Quality Improvement Organization
- Military and Veterans Administration
- Nurses
- Pharmacies
- Philanthropies/Foundations
- Physicians and Physician Practices
- Public Health Agencies
- State Primary Care Association(s)
- State Medicaid Agency
- Tribes
- Universities
- Vendors
- Visiting Nurse Association

Figure 2-8: List of Potential Stakeholders

this book, we continually refer to the importance of stakeholder engagement and participation. There are basic principles for stakeholder engagement and participation that you must keep in mind throughout your HIE formation efforts and on into your operational stage. These are summarized for you in Figure 2-9.

Develop Your Communication Plan

A solid communication plan is a key component in successfully engaging and retaining the interest of your stakeholders. Developing a good communication plan with effective methods and messages tailored to your different stakeholder groups is one of the keystones to your success.

- Understand your community.
- Engage the right stakeholders.
- Engage your stakeholders early and often.
- Understand that how you interact with different stakeholder segments will change over time.
- Understand that what your stakeholders value will change throughout the stages of the HIE life cycle.
- Check that your organization's core principles accurately reflect your stakeholders' values.
- Adopt organizational policies that will make it easy for your stakeholders to maintain their trust.
- Measure your success based upon how well you are meeting your stakeholders key wants and needs.
- Validate that you are meeting their key wants and needs by asking them directly.

Figure 2-9: Key Principles for Stakeholder Participation

> **Caution**
> If it does not feel like you are over communicating, you are probably not communicating enough.

Remember, your communication plan is a living, dynamic plan. It will, and should, change regularly. You will constantly be updating and enhancing your plan as you reach major milestones, seek to involve additional people and organizations in your efforts, require additional community input, or seek additional funding. The status of your communication plan should be on every meeting agenda and openly discussed to ensure that your efforts are coordinated. Be sure that the communication plan and its activities accurately reflect the progress that you make and—even more importantly—the feedback that you receive from your various interactions with stakeholders continuously informs your planning efforts.

Your initial community assessment provides you with a good indication of the different stakeholder groups in your community and their perspectives on HIE. Various stakeholder groups require different types of messages and your level of communication with those stakeholder groups will vary, depending on where you are in your planning efforts. This is typical in change management projects. And it is important to always remember that forming an HIE is a change management project—albeit one with a substantial technical component.

If it does not feel like you are over communicating, you are probably not communicating enough. This is certainly true when it comes to forming and operating HIEs. Gina Perez, from the Delaware Health Information Network (DHIN), emphasizes "...inviting everyone to the table. Talk to people and find out what HIE means to them." Many of the successful HIEs use multiple communication channels such as newspapers, public meetings, and presentations to civic clubs and religious organizations. Others recommend individual meetings with key stakeholders to make sure their concerns are addressed.

Developing a solid communication plan is important because it helps you (1) think through and determine what you want to accomplish; (2) understand the environment in which you are operating; (3) understand to whom you will target your messages; and (4) hone your messages so they are both crisp and relevant to each audience. The plan will also ensure that messages from your organization are consistent and that everyone on the team is on the same page in their communications. It is vitally important not to confuse your community!

Steps to Develop the Communication Plan

One of the first things you need to do is assess your needs for communication. You must identify your target audience(s); understand your communication goals and objectives; and create your initial key messages.

For example, initially your communication may be to inform and educate the community about HIE. Later, you may be seeking their input or communicating your accomplishments.

Your audience, goals, and messages for specific stakeholder groups may change over time. It is critical that you send messages that resonate with your target audiences.

Remember: Everyone in your community listens to radio station *WII FM*—"What's In It For Me?" Make sure you tell them!

Different target audiences react differently to different communication methods. While the "boomers" may respond well to emails and even text messaging, GenX, GenY, and Millennials rely heavily on tweets, Facebook, and other forms of social networking. It is important to create strategies for reaching each of your target audiences.

Be diligent about integrating your communication plan into your overall planning activities. Actively seek out opportunities to publicize your accomplishments and seek input from your stakeholders. Regular communication is one of the best methods you can use to keep your stakeholders engaged in your HIE efforts.

Developing a solid, effective communication plan involves both art and science. Consider bringing in someone experienced with communication planning. Figure 2-10 summarizes the steps to developing an effective and dynamic communication plan.

There are many excellent resources available to help you develop a good communication plan, and we list many of them at the end of this chapter. One example of a good (and no cost) resource is the HHS Health IT Consumer Education and Engagement website.[1] This is a good source for locating education plans and materials for consumers and contains resources, a planning guide, materials, and examples of communication plans. Figure 2-11 provides some tips for good communication.

Reaching Beyond Your Immediate Community

You will also want to communicate outside of your immediate community, particularly with your State Designated Entity and Regional Extension Center.

❏ 1. Assess your needs for communication.
        a. With whom do you need to communicate?
        b. What do you need to tell them or ask them?
        c. Do you want something from them?
        d. Are you informing, educating, seeking input or buy-in, hoping
            to obtain funding, or motivating people to participate?

❏ 2. Identify your target audiences.

❏ 3. Develop your key messages.

❏ 4. Create strategies to reach your target audiences.

❏ 5. Identify the timing for your various types of communication
        activities.

❏ 6. Begin thinking about the actual process of communicating:
        a. Various channels
        b. Frequency
        c. Media types

❏ 7. Determine who your spokespersons will be. They may
        change depending on the stakeholder group and where you
        are in the process.

❏ 8. Integrate communication into your overall HIE development
        plan.

❏ 9. Make communication a discussion item on every meeting
        agenda.

Figure 2-10: Checklist—Developing the Initial Communication Plan

- Communicate with stakeholders and continually evaluate their
  commitment level.
- Provide recognition for key stakeholders within the community.
- Keep stakeholders informed of what's happening.
- Build stakeholder communication into all of your processes.

Figure 2-11: Tips for Communication

Engage with Your State Designated Entity for HIE

Under HITECH, State Designated Entities are the organizations that receive federal money to assist the HIE movement by providing a statewide HIE infrastructure. Chapter 1, *The HIE Landscape*, includes a more in-depth discussion of State Designated Entities. One of the primary goals of the State Designated Entity is "to promote the use of health IT to improve health care quality and efficiency through the authorized and secure electronic exchange and use of health information."[2]

Communicate with your state's State Designated Entity early in your planning efforts. Get to know the people involved. Let them know of your intent to form an HIE. Understand the types of resources they can provide so you can coordinate your efforts with state-led efforts.

The individuals from your HIE who are assigned to interact with the State Designated Entity should be knowledgeable about your project and able to communicate effectively with both the State Designated Entity representatives and your committee. They should be able to solicit support for your activities, effectively communicate your progress to the State Designated Entity, and provide you with information related to the prospective and available resources of the State Designated Entity. You should consider your State Designated Entity a key stakeholder in your HIE's success, so engaging and interacting with the State Designated Entity is a key element of your communication plan. Each State Designated Entity is approaching their formation a bit differently. They are sensitive to the norms, cultures, and laws within their states.

Engage with Your Local Health Information Technology Regional Extension Center

Under HITECH, the Regional Extension Centers are charged with assisting providers in implementing EMRs (electronic medical records) and achieving *Meaningful Use*. One of the key components required to obtain meaningful use incentives from CMS is the actual exchange of health information. Meaningful use and the Regional Extension Centers are discussed in more detail in Chapter 1, *The HIE Landscape*. Since the Regional Extension Centers are responsible for helping eligible providers connect electronically—and then ensuring that those providers achieve meaningful use—they can be a useful resource for the HIE in helping to reach out to the provider community. Become acquainted with the people running the Regional Extension Centers in your area. You should also consider the Regional Extension Center a key stakeholder in your HIE's success.

It is important to work with both your State Designated Entity and the Regional Extension Center to ensure that you are aware of both the potential funding and the resource assistance they have to offer. Seek to leverage their capabilities. Ensure that you are not duplicating efforts. And, by working closely with them, you can gain access to "motivated" stakeholders in your community and potential future customers.

Congratulations. You are on your way.

In the next chapter, we discuss getting further commitment from your stakeholders, forming your Steering Committee and creating your HIE's vision and mission.

CHAPTER SUMMARY

In this chapter we provided an overview of the five stages of the HIE lifecycle and the five domains that we believe represent the work areas for developing an HIE.

We discussed how, in the Initiation Stage, the Exploratory Committee begins to assess the potential of an HIE in the community. This committee should gain an understanding of the community from several perspectives. Once you reach a decision to move forward, you enter the Formation Stage.

We discussed how identification of, and continuous engagement with your stakeholders is essential to your success. This means that you continuously solicit their input and respond to their needs. Therefore, the communication plan plays a key role throughout your HIE life cycle and is paramount in maintaining stakeholder engagement which, in turn, is a requirement for your future sustainability.

Lastly, we discussed involving the State Designated Entity and Regional Extension Center in your planning efforts. Coordinating with them, and using the resources they offer, can help you throughout your planning efforts.

When you complete the activities in this chapter, you will have:
- An understanding of the five stages of the HIE life cycle;
- An understanding of the five domains of HIE formation;
- Formed an exploratory committee;
- Assessed your community at a high level;
- Identified key stakeholders and have begun working with them;
- Initiated development and use of the communication plan;
- Engaged with your State Designated Entity;
- Engaged with your Regional Extension Center; and
- Entered the Formation Stage.

CASE STUDIES
Indiana Health Information Technology, Inc. (IHIT)

David Johnson, President and CEO, BioCrossroads

Creating Indiana's State Designated Entity for the State HIE Collaborative Agreement Program:

As the HITECH programs were being developed and rolled out, Indiana wanted to ensure a coordinated approach that would benefit the entire state. On behalf of the state and the private-sector HIOs, BioCrossroads convened a group representing the HIOs in the state, the universities, and other interested parties to create a not-for-profit entity, IHIT, Inc., which was formed through the participation of all key stakeholders in the state. The approach is to source contracts to the HIOs within the state to provide the required services.

Indiana is unique in that the state, under its constitution, is prohibited from issuing direct debt and was, for many years, restricted from making investments in any form of corporate securities. As a result, and also through a strong tradition of public-private partnerships, the state is very experienced in working in collaboration with private entities to establish 501(c)3 public-private entities to administer initiatives.

An experienced not-for-profit organization and neutral third party, BioCrossroads, was tasked to be the facilitator and neutral broker of this effort and took the lead in applying for the ARRA State Health Information Exchange Collaborative Agreement Program grant funds. BioCrossroads then drove the creation on behalf of the state of the operating 501(c)3 entity, IHIT, Inc.

According to David Johnson, President and CEO, BioCrossroads, the convening organization, the approach Indiana took was based on the principle of bringing the best experience and expertise to the table and linking them together. The neutrality of having a third party facilitate the formation of the organization enabled all of the involved organizations to discuss their perspectives openly and coordinate as the state team. The process was designed so that all stakeholders had a voice in IHIT's formation and all felt included.

State of Michigan

Beth Nagel, HIT Coordinator, Michigan Department of Community Health

In Michigan, as of this writing, there is not yet a formal State Designated Entity. However, there has already been a great deal of effort put into stakeholder engagement. According to Beth Nagel, HIT Coordinator for Michigan, they have used a collaborative approach to convene an extensive network of interested stakeholders. Their approach is to build a statewide HIE by leveraging the local sub-state HIEs that are currently functioning or forming. According to Nagel, Michigan is "modeling the statewide approach after the NHIN."

Based on Michigan's experience in convening statewide stakeholder groups, Nagel recommends the following:

- It is imperative to have an open and transparent process. Nagel says, "This can be a 'messy' process, since everyone is allowed their input, but it is a necessary process and the right thing for building trust."
- Take your time and build that trust.
- Do not be afraid of making mistakes, as long as you learn from them.
- Let your stakeholders express themselves—this can be an excellent opportunity to learn from mistakes and go back to the drawing board and start over, if necessary.
- Talk to your stakeholders about finances often.
- Communicate, communicate, communicate—get people involved early.

Arizona Health-e Connection (AzHeC)

Brad Tritle, Executive Director, Arizona Health-e Connection

Arizona Health-e Connection (AzHeC) engages its stakeholders on numerous levels, seeking to understand stakeholder needs for education and direction and then finding the best solutions to meet those needs. AzHeC is in constant communication with stakeholders, and this process helps the organization identify value-added activities they can offer.

AzHeC hosts an annual summit, holds educational webinars, and provides on-site presentations to keep current stakeholders engaged, as well as to bring on new, relevant stakeholders. AzHeC's e-mail distribution list is 1,400+ contacts across the Western region.

To keep and add stakeholders AzHeC maintains strong relationships with Healthcare Information and Management Systems Society (HIMSS) and American Health Information Management Association (AHIMA) state chapters by speaking at their meetings and co-sponsoring events; providing CMEs to practitioners in conjunction with Medical and Osteopathic Societies, American College of Physicians, Nurse Practitioner Council, and Arizona State Association of Physician Assistants; and finally, AzHeC works collaboratively with its stakeholders and encourages them to share their ideas.

Delaware Health Information Network (DHIN)

Gina Bianco Perez, Executive Director, DHIN

Delaware has been very successful with stakeholder engagement. According to Gina Perez, Executive Director, DHIN, it's important to recognize at the beginning that some people may not be ready for health information exchange. She recommends listening to their concerns and addressing them. Everyone needs to be heard.

Perez recommends the following ways to keep stakeholders participating:
- Conduct meetings that are meaningful to your stakeholders.
- Continue to invite stakeholders to your meetings.
- Show success and others will come.

RESOURCES

HIE Educational Tools. Technology CEO Council. 2005. http://himss.org/ASP/topics_FocusDynamic. asp?faid=141. Accessed September, 2010.

E-Health Readiness Guide. http://www.techceocouncil.org. Accessed September, 2010.

Department of Health & Human Services. State Health Information Exchange Cooperative Agreement Program. http://healthit.hhs.gov/portal/server.pt?open=512&objID=1336&mode=2&cached =true. Accessed November, 2009.

Department of Health & Human Services. HITECH Priority Grants Program: State Health Information Exchange Cooperative Agreement Program. Facts at a Glance. http://healthit.hhs.gov/portal/server.pt? open=512&objID=1333&parentname=CommunityPage&parentid=47&mode=2&in_hi_userid=11113& cached=true#. Accessed September, 2010.

W. K. Kellogg Foundation. Communications Toolkit. http://www.wkkf.org/default.aspx?tabid=75&CID= 385&NID=61&LanguageID=0. Accessed September, 2010.

Health Information Security & Privacy Collaboration (HISPC). Provider Education Toolkit (PET) Explained. Posted June 9, 2009. http://healthit.hhs.gov/portal/server.pt/gateway/PTARGS_0_10741_ 875062_0_0_18/PET_Workshop.pdf. Accessed October, 2010.

Health Information Security & Privacy Collaboration (HISPC). Provider Education Toolkit (PET). Posted June 9, 2009. http://www.secure4health.org/. Accessed October, 2010.

eHealth4NY.org. Resources. http://www.ehealth4ny.org/resources.html. Accessed September, 2010.

Brooklyn Health Information Exchange (BHIX). Patient Educational Fact Sheet. http://bhix.org/ downloads/BHIX_EducationalBrochure.pdf. Accessed September, 2010.

American Hospital Association (AHA). Health Information Exchange Projects: What Hospitals and Health Systems Need to Know. 2006. http://www.aha.org/aha/content/2006/pdf/AHARHIOfinal.pdf. Accessed September, 2010.

REFERENCES

1. Department of Health & Human Services, Office of the National Coordinator for Health Information Technology. Consumer Education and Engagement. http://healthit.hhs.gov/portal/server.pt?open=512&objID=1280&PageID=16051&mode=2&cached=true. Accessed April, 2010.

2. Department of Health & Human Services, Office of the National Coordinator for Health Information Technology. State Health Information Exchange Cooperative Agreement Program, Funding Opportunity Announcement, 2009; 15. http://healthit.hhs.gov/portal/server.pt/gateway/PTARGS_0_10741_888442_0_0_18/FOA_State%20Health%20Information%20Exchange%20Cooperative%20Agreement%20Program_Sept3_updated%20funding%20formula.doc. Accessed April, 2010.

CHAPTER 3

Navigating Your Early Stage Formation

Strive to form the kind of organization in which
your stakeholders will want to participate.

INTRODUCTION

Now begins the intense effort of forming your HIE. You completed the Initiation Stage and moved into the Formation Stage when you determined that there was both sufficient interest and need in your community to form an HIE.

In this chapter, we describe what you should do to transition your Exploratory Committee into your Steering Committee. The Steering Committee is the group of people who will guide your efforts until you establish your formal Board of Directors. We also discuss what you need to do to identify early funding sources; identify and engage expert assistance; and begin to develop your strategic plan—specifically how to create your organization's Vision and Mission Statements. Of course, all of this is done with the active and open participation of your key stakeholders.

As you begin your early formation efforts, it is helpful to keep in mind some of the characteristics that describe successful HIEs. The key to success rests in forming the kind of organization in which your stakeholders will want to actively participate. Figure 3-1 summarizes the characteristics that, in our experience, are common to most successful HIEs.

FORMING THE STEERING COMMITTEE

Now that you are committed to moving forward with your HIE's formation, it is important to form your Steering Committee. The Steering Committee can be known by a variety of names—Advisory Committee, Advisory Board, or others. What is important is that this is the initial group that will actually lead your formation efforts. This step begins to formalize your efforts. The Steering Committee sets the tone for your success.

Dick Thompson, Executive Director/CEO of Quality Health Network in Grand Junction, Colorado, suggests specific ways to set the tone of your efforts:

1. Establish the altruistic motives for the organization. You have to have something everyone agrees is worth doing or improving.

- Your guiding principles are in alignment with the stakeholders' values, and your community's culture and norms.
- The people forming your HIE are trusted and trustworthy in the eyes of your stakeholders.
- The HIE provides open and transparent governance that builds and continues to foster trust.
- Stakeholders trust that privacy will be maintained by the HIE.
- The HIE provides the services that stakeholders have said they want.
- The fees charged are aligned with the value that participants believe they are receiving.

Figure 3-1: Attributes of a Successful HIE

2. Pick specific items to deliver. Do it in small steps. Do something, but don't try to boil the ocean. After you are successful at one thing, find something else to do and do it well.
3. Set expectations at a level that will allow you to win and that can be met and exceeded.
4. Plan for mistakes and allow room for recovery; it's not easy. Telling people it's easy to build the HIE is a MISTAKE.
5. Identify the three things that are important to your stakeholders—and then deliver them.
6. Recruit and retain the best people you can find; ones that can communicate and LISTEN.
7. Be confident. **This is doable.** Stay the course.

Establishing the Steering Committee is an important step in HIE formation. It is this group that serves as the initial governance and management body for the formation of your HIE. In some cases, early stage HIE efforts have opted to designate a Board rather than a Steering Committee. That may or may not be the right thing to do in your situation. The timing for moving from a Steering Committee to a formal Board depends upon your status as a legal entity—whether or not you immediately form a legal entity or there is a sponsoring organization that can "incubate" your effort while you form—and the norms and culture of your community.

The Steering Committee has the responsibility for governance and community outreach for the HIE formation project until a formal Board is designated. Once the Board is established, this responsibility moves to the Board.

To ensure that you identify and recruit the right people for the Steering Committee, it's important to understand the initial roles, responsibilities, and expectations of Steering Committee members. Whom you select to be on the Steering Committee is determined by individuals' passion for HIE, the skills and resources they can bring, their ability to commit time and resources to your effort, their ability to collaborate, and their willingness to put the community's need above their own interests.

The Steering Committee is responsible for getting your project moving. There is a lot of work to do. The following are some of their responsibilities:

- Lead the formation efforts.
- Promote the concept of HIE within your community.
- Build trust among the stakeholders and with your larger community.
- Coordinate the work of the various workgroups that you will be establishing.
- Approve recommendations from the workgroups and ensure that they are implemented.
- Create and implement your plan to establish the HIE.
- Create and manage the initial version of the budget.

A Steering Committee should include people who are opinion leaders and can effectively communicate both the value and the needs of your HIE formation efforts. As with the Exploratory Committee, you want to add people to the Steering Committee who are perceived as leaders in the healthcare community, as well as in the community at large. The Steering Committee should be comprised of people who can see the big picture, who believe in the cause, and who are able to manage the activities required to achieve it. Think about adding people with specific expertise or access to key resources. Make sure you have a good mix of skills and personalities on this committee. Avoid the mistake of filling the Steering Committee with all of the same type of people, such as technical experts, physicians, lawyers, etc. Find the people who will provide the well-rounded leadership necessary to make your HIE a success.

It is essential to include at least one representative from the provider community, specifically, someone who is passionate about making this happen, someone with the skills to communicate the idea to others in the provider community and beyond to motivate them to participate. Other individuals to consider approaching are those with hands-on knowledge of clinical care, representatives of the other key stakeholder groups, and interested consumers.

You will need to get commitment from the people who serve on the Steering Committee. Many of those on your Exploratory Committee will meet the criteria to become Steering Committee members and will agree to continue to participate. Others may not be the right fit for the Steering Committee, or they may not be able to make the required commitment of time. That's okay. Members of the Exploratory Committee who do not become members of the Steering Committee are still valuable to your organization. There is still a place where they may stay engaged in the project. Consider them as you look to staff the various workgroups that we mention later in this chapter. The important thing is to get the right people on the Steering Committee.

Every effort needs a leader, and your Steering Committee is no exception. Identify a person who will be responsible for leading your efforts. Most likely, this will be a voluntary position at this stage. Choose someone who the community and the other Steering Committee members view as a leader. Optimally, this person will have a natural talent for leadership, a passion for your HIE efforts, excellent public speaking skills, and the ability to motivate others. This person should be a *leader,* not a manager.

While conducting interviews for this book, we repeatedly heard how important it is, early on, to get people involved who are passionate about forming the HIE *for the benefit of the community*. They must be able to look beyond their own organization's

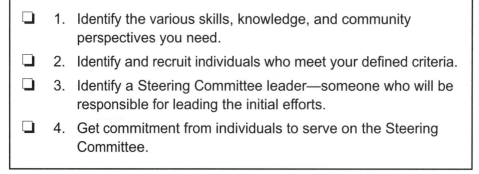

1. Identify the various skills, knowledge, and community perspectives you need.
2. Identify and recruit individuals who meet your defined criteria.
3. Identify a Steering Committee leader—someone who will be responsible for leading the initial efforts.
4. Get commitment from individuals to serve on the Steering Committee.

Figure 3-2: Checklist—Forming a Steering Committee

best interests and work in the best interests of the larger community. There is no time, and no room, for individual agendas at this point. This is hard work, and you need both passion and a focus on the community to keep this effort moving forward.

Figure 3-2 provides a checklist of some of the activities to include as you go about forming your Steering Committee.

Ongoing Responsibilities of the Steering Committee

Establishing the Steering Committee is just the beginning. There is still much more work to do. The Steering Committee and, when formed, the Board, is responsible for guiding and overseeing several workgroups. These are the groups that will develop and recommend plans to the Steering Committee related to specific domains of the HIE. Figure 3-3 shows the five domains for which workgroups need to be formed.

As part of your HIE formation effort, each domain workgroup has specific tasks to perform and milestones to reach. These tasks are best accomplished by people with domain-specific expertise and experience. Now is the time to think about how you will staff these workgroups. Think about and describe the required skills needed for each of the groups. Think about how they will function. Identify and contact individuals who have the appropriate skills and experience to help you in these domains, and determine if they are willing and able to help.

In contrast to Steering Committee members, the people the Steering Committee recruits for the individual workgroups should have an in-depth knowledge of, and experience in, the specific subject area the workgroup is charged to address. Their job is to develop the details necessary for your formation planning. In Chapter 4, *Establish a Formal Organizational Governance Structure*, we go into more detail on specific objectives for each workgroup.

- Stakeholder Engagement & Participation
- Business & Finance
- Governance
- Privacy
- Technology & Security

Figure 3-3: Workgroup Domains

INITIAL ORGANIZATIONAL VISION AND MISSION

It is important to define your vision and mission early in your formation process. When you have a vision that is inspirational and a mission that is motivational, you have a solid framework for the many subsequent decisions you will need to make. Well-constructed Vision and Mission Statements ensure that all those involved in establishing the HIE are in concert and are working toward a common, understandable goal. Devore Culver, Executive Director and CEO, HealthInfoNet, recommends building a vision that allows the various perspectives to share some "common space." While there may be areas of disagreement, "Work HARD on what's common, and acknowledge areas of disagreement."

Your Vision Statement is an inspirational description of the future state. Your vision emphasizes the future—what you want to help bring about. The mission of your organization describes the fundamental purpose for which you exist. It connects your present with your future. While the Mission Statement should stretch you, it also needs to fall within the realm of being achievable. Your Mission Statement is an essential tool for communicating to the community and stakeholders what your group is attempting to accomplish—and why. We provide several examples of Vision and Mission Statements in Appendix A.

Creating Your Vision and Mission Statements

As described in Chapter 2, *Getting Started*, when you held your Exploratory Committee meetings, some of the areas you discussed were your views of the future—when your HIE would become a reality. You talked about what you hope to accomplish by forming the HIE; what you want the HIE to become; how your community will benefit by using the services and capabilities your HIE provides; and the role that the HIE will play in achieving that future. These discussions were the beginning of your Vision and Mission Statements. Check the notes that you took at those early meetings. You can build on those ideas.

> Your Vision and Mission Statements should meet these key criteria.
>
> - Clearly communicate what you care about
> - Inspire passion and action

Often the vision and mission are developed concurrently. In our experience, this is an iterative process, and the ideas you generate for one will, in turn, feed ideas for and help shape the other. Throughout this book, we continually urge you to go directly to your stakeholders for their input and opinions. This is definitely one of those times. Defining your vision and mission should be a community effort and should be built by consensus. Typically, you start by brainstorming with some of the early ideas from your Exploratory Committee meetings.

A key component in creating your vision and mission is ensuring that you are developing a vision and mission that is truly in sync, not only with your Steering Committee, but, more importantly, with your

> You must achieve buy-in on the vision and mission by your key stakeholders before you move forward.

broader community of key stakeholders. As previously mentioned, the best way to do this is to ask them directly. You can do this through focus groups, surveys, and targeted townhall-type meetings. Use this as a communication opportunity to strengthen your community foundation. This is an early and important component of your communication plan.

Developing Your Vision Statement

Your vision is exactly that. It is your vision of the desired future as it relates to healthcare and the role that HIE will play. Developing your vision is a creative process that involves brainstorming and a lot of input and discussion. Your vision should be far-reaching and aspirational.

While your vision describes what you want your future to be, it is important to remember that the Vision Statement is not a description of action steps. Rather, it describes your desired future state and serves as a clear guide for choosing both your current and future courses of action. See Figure 3-4 for an example.

There are many examples of HIE Vision Statements provided in Appendix A. Figure 3-5 lists the steps you may want to use as you create your Vision Statement.

Developing Your Mission Statement

> Your mission should inspire passion and action in your stakeholders.

The Mission Statement should (1) be based on your vision; (2) be concise; and (3) be developed from your stakeholders' perspectives. It links your vision of the future with the day-to-day realities of your community.

The following questions will be helpful as you develop your Mission Statement. A good Mission Statement clearly and concisely answers all three questions.

1. *What do we do?*
   Answer this question in terms of what stakeholder and community needs you fulfill with your efforts. State the needs you will address and the capabilities you will provide to the community.
2. *How do we do it?*
   The answer to this question should reflect the actual service or products that you will provide. It needs to fit with the needs you are addressing.
3. *For whom do we do it?*
   The answer to this question helps you focus on the specific population(s) whose needs you are addressing. Define your target: who will use, and benefit from, your services?

The widespread use of the health information exchange dramatically improves the quality of healthcare delivery and lowers healthcare costs in the Central State region.

Figure 3-4: Example Vision Statement

❏ 1. Determine whom to involve.
      Consider the Steering Committee members, key stakeholders, and other influential community leaders.

❏ 2. Brainstorm for words that describe the future you want to see.

❏ 3. Identify and agree on the important attributes of that future state.

❏ 4. Consolidate the attributes and create trial statements.

❏ 5. Discuss and adjust the statements until you reach consensus on the Vision Statement.

❏ 6. Document and communicate the vision.

Figure 3-5: Steps to Creating the Vision Statement

The Mission Statement does not need to be all-encompassing at this time. It is okay if it is initially very focused. As your HIE matures, you can expand your mission to include more services and a broader stakeholder base. Figure 3-6 provides one example of a good initial Mission Statement.

Once you have a good draft of your Vision and Mission Statements, you need to test them. Your mission should inspire passion in you and your stakeholders. Does it excite you? Does it clearly and concisely state your purpose? Your mission should clearly communicate your reason for being to those who are not directly involved in your efforts. We provide examples of HIE Mission Statements in Appendix A. Figure 3-7 recaps steps you can use in creating your Mission Statement.

We have found that developing your vision and mission can best be accomplished using a neutral facilitator who has the skills and techniques to guide the process. While you can accomplish this without outside guidance, there is a danger that not all perspectives will be aired or that one person's or one group's own agenda might dominate the discussion. An experienced outside facilitator typically has the tools, methodologies, and skills to help you develop strong, relevant Vision and Mission Statements. This person can ensure that all perspectives are voiced and that your committee can reach consensus and buy-in on the organization's vision and mission. If not everyone can agree on your vision and mission, keep working on them. Figure 3-8 provides a summary of the steps you need to take to develop your Vision and Mission Statements.

The Central State HIE will provide the resources and guidance to improve the quality of healthcare delivery and lower healthcare costs. We will do this by developing and providing the core services and capabilities required to manage and appropriately exchange health information in the Central State region.

Figure 3-6: Example Mission Statement

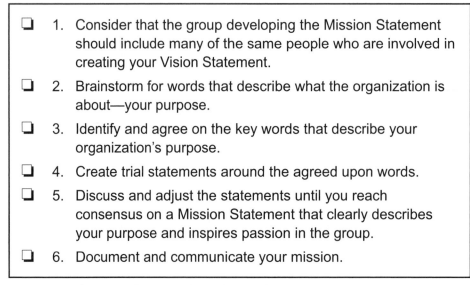

❑   1.   Consider that the group developing the Mission Statement should include many of the same people who are involved in creating your Vision Statement.

❑   2.   Brainstorm for words that describe what the organization is about—your purpose.

❑   3.   Identify and agree on the key words that describe your organization's purpose.

❑   4.   Create trial statements around the agreed upon words.

❑   5.   Discuss and adjust the statements until you reach consensus on a Mission Statement that clearly describes your purpose and inspires passion in the group.

❑   6.   Document and communicate your mission.

Figure 3-7: Steps to Creating the Mission Statement

❑   1.   Identify the key people to involve in developing your organization's vision and mission.

❑   2.   Create the HIE vision.

❑   3.   Develop the HIE mission.

❑   4.   Reach consensus and buy-in for the vision and mission.

❑   5.   Document the vision and mission.

❑   6.   Review the vision and mission with all relevant stakeholders and incorporate their feedback.

❑   7.   Have the steering committee formally approve the Vision and Mission Statements.

❑   8.   Communicate the vision and mission.

Figure 3-8: Developing Your Vision and Mission

You will revisit, review, and reread your Vision and Mission Statements on a regular basis. You should do this not only to keep yourself focused on the scope of what you want to achieve, but also to ensure that your mission remains appropriate given your changing environment and circumstances.

In Chapter 5, *Creating Your Strategic Plan*, and Chapter 6, *Your Business Plan Defines How Delivering Value Drives Your Sustainability*, we discuss how you bring your vision to reality by beginning to execute your mission. You do this through creating your strategic plan and your business plan. These plans include objectives, strategic approaches, and specific initiatives. They are all built upon, and serve and support, your Mission Statement.

We cannot emphasize enough the importance of stakeholder engagement as you develop your Vision and Mission Statements. We have repeatedly found that successful HIEs have had solid stakeholder involvement in these early efforts.

According to Laura Adams, President and CEO of the Rhode Island Quality Institute, "Stakeholder engagement is the key to everything."

LETTERS OF COMMITMENT

As we mentioned earlier, you are about to embark on a large community-wide change effort. In many cases, you are building an organization from scratch. It is vitally important to have early and visible commitment from your stakeholders. One approach we have seen in many successful HIE efforts is to request a signed letter of commitment from each member of your newly formed Steering Committee. If you can also obtain letters of commitment from others in your community, in addition to those from the Steering Committee members, that will help strengthen your chances for success. At this point you are only asking for their support in forming (and hopefully one day using) the HIE.

This formal recognition by your community leaders that HIE should be pursued for the benefit of your community is an essential early step in developing stakeholder engagement and participation. Obtaining letters of commitment shows that there is sufficient understanding and support for HIE in the community and that the key stakeholders will publicly commit to the effort. This is important because it is a demonstration of their willingness to publicly and formally take action to support the formation of your HIE.

The letter should be a simple, direct letter of support. Figure 3-9 provides an example of an early letter of commitment.

The ongoing process of building stakeholder engagement and support continues as you expand the list of active stakeholders. Communicate with them the importance of HIE. Early on, it is important to identify those people in your healthcare community, and your community at large, who are influential and who are opinion leaders. These are the people you need to focus on and gain their early support.

Do not expect, at this stage, to have the committed support of all the key stakeholders in your community. However, you should ensure that your support is both broad and sufficient enough to continue with your HIE activities. Do not stop your efforts at communication, though, when you have the initial set of letters from your key stakeholders. Using your communication plan activities, continue to solicit letters of support and commitment from additional key people and organizations throughout your formation efforts. Keep building your stakeholder support and your credibility base.

Figure 3–10 suggests steps you need to take to obtain these letters of commitment.

EARLY FUNDING

It is never too soon to think about sources of funding for your efforts. Once you receive signed letters of commitment, a request for funding is a natural follow-on activity. Of course you need to be able to develop and present an initial plan describing how you will provide value to your stakeholders before you begin to solicit funding. It is also

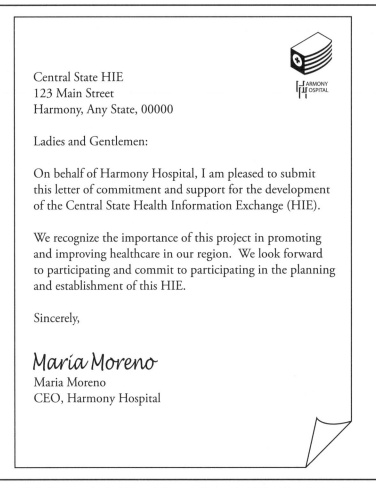

Central State HIE
123 Main Street
Harmony, Any State, 00000

Ladies and Gentlemen:

On behalf of Harmony Hospital, I am pleased to submit
this letter of commitment and support for the development
of the Central State Health Information Exchange (HIE).

We recognize the importance of this project in promoting
and improving healthcare in our region. We look forward
to participating and commit to participating in the planning
and establishment of this HIE.

Sincerely,

Maria Moreno
Maria Moreno
CEO, Harmony Hospital

Figure 3-9: Example Letter of Commitment. *Note:* The federal government
required letters of support to be submitted with all of the state proposals for the
State Health Information Exchange Cooperative Agreement Program grants and
for the HIT Regional Extension Center grant applications. Those letters might
provide you with specific working options and the names of specific individuals
and organizations that could support your HIE.

important to present a clearly identified purpose for the upfront funds you are requesting, such as to contract with a consultant to bring in the expertise and intellectual capital that will help you get started, or to provide funding for initial staff. This plan supports your initial funding requests.

In addition to the obvious benefits of having money in the bank, securing early
funding from key stakeholders takes them to the next level of commitment. Both our
experience, and leading practices, show that it is important to get stakeholders to invest
financially early on in your efforts. The amounts requested do not have to be large sums,
they can be in the $5,000–$10,000 range, depending on your anticipated needs and
what is appropriate for your community.

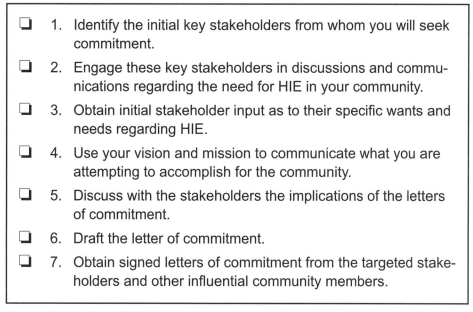

1. Identify the initial key stakeholders from whom you will seek commitment.

2. Engage these key stakeholders in discussions and communications regarding the need for HIE in your community.

3. Obtain initial stakeholder input as to their specific wants and needs regarding HIE.

4. Use your vision and mission to communicate what you are attempting to accomplish for the community.

5. Discuss with the stakeholders the implications of the letters of commitment.

6. Draft the letter of commitment.

7. Obtain signed letters of commitment from the targeted stakeholders and other influential community members.

Figure 3-10: Checklist—Obtaining Letters of Commitment

We have found that early stakeholder financial commitment can be positively associated with the growth and success of an HIE. The opposite—little or no stakeholder financial investment—can be similarly correlated to a lack of success of HIE efforts.

We have not found any solid evidence about whether the level of stakeholder buy-in for the perceived value that HIE will provide leads to the level of investment, or whether the level of investment leads to more attention and active participation. However, we do believe that it is the early perception of value that helps drive stakeholder participation.

The process of soliciting funds from key stakeholders provides a good opportunity to, once again, gather input from your stakeholders. Do they believe that you are on the right track? Do they believe that you have been listening to them and incorporating their input?

To jump-start your efforts, we recommend that you identify one or two influential stakeholders who are willing, and able, to make a financial commitment. Help them to 'lead by example' and get their help in convincing others that this is the right thing to do.

Remember, the contribution of cash to the HIE effort is tangible proof that stakeholders see enough potential value in forming your HIE that they are willing to invest financially. It also adds credence to their earlier letter of commitment.

The willingness of stakeholders to contribute financially helps you identify those stakeholders who are actively willing to provide resources to help move your effort forward versus others who are not willing to invest and, thus, may only be 'interested observers.' Knowing the level of commitment of each of your stakeholders helps you determine who may be viable candidates to become Board members in the future.

Do not be shy about asking for funding. This worthy endeavor will benefit the entire community. When you ask for funding, communicate what you are doing, why

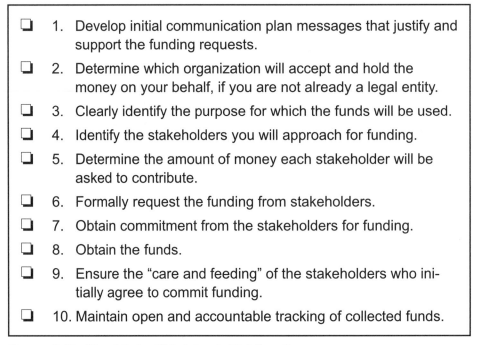

❏   1. Develop initial communication plan messages that justify and support the funding requests.

❏   2. Determine which organization will accept and hold the money on your behalf, if you are not already a legal entity.

❏   3. Clearly identify the purpose for which the funds will be used.

❏   4. Identify the stakeholders you will approach for funding.

❏   5. Determine the amount of money each stakeholder will be asked to contribute.

❏   6. Formally request the funding from stakeholders.

❏   7. Obtain commitment from the stakeholders for funding.

❏   8. Obtain the funds.

❏   9. Ensure the "care and feeding" of the stakeholders who initially agree to commit funding.

❏   10. Maintain open and accountable tracking of collected funds.

Figure 3-11: Checklist—Obtaining Initial Funding

you are doing it, and how the funds will be used. As you develop your initial fundraising approach, we recommend that you find examples from other similar not-for-profit organizations in your community to learn how they raised their initial funding. There may also be fundraising expertise among your Steering Committee members. Use the expertise and existing community networks of your committed stakeholders to obtain your early funding.

Designate a person with the responsibility to accurately track and report the receipt and expenditure of the funds. This effort requires an open, transparent, and accurate reporting and tracking of funds. Remember, you are accountable for your financial situation from the beginning. Begin early to build credibility and trust in your organization by being fiscally responsible and transparent. Figure 3-11 lists some of the steps to consider as you seek early funding.

ENGAGING HIE FORMATION SUBJECT MATTER EXPERTS

Initially, most, if not all, of your Steering Committee members will be volunteers. Most likely they will have little prior experience with forming an HIE. Our experience shows that there is no "silver bullet" or shortcut to forming an HIE. Nothing takes the place of going through all the steps with your community. You need to build their trust and support, and this takes time. However, it is helpful to draw from lessons learned from prior successful (and unsuccessful) HIE efforts.

It is important, if not essential, to seek outside resources as you develop your HIE. A competent subject matter expert (SME), with experience in guiding others in forming an HIE, is an invaluable asset to your efforts. This person, or firm, can bring knowledge of the lessons they and others have learned, as well as the necessary skills and expertise in methods and tools, to help speed your efforts. Understanding and having experience with what has worked—and what has not worked—for other similar efforts can significantly improve your efficiency and effectiveness as you form your HIE.

Assess Your Need

A good place to start in assessing the type of external resources you need to bring in is to first understand the full range of expertise and skills that you need to form your HIE. These skills include an understanding of the HIE landscape; experience in community organization and stakeholder engagement; an understanding of how to build an organization from the ground up; experience in creating HIE-specific governance; an understanding of how to develop your financial model; in-depth understanding of the privacy rules; and expertise in the use of health IT.

Once you have a good grasp of the various areas of expertise required, look first to your own Steering Committee for resources. Determine the level of expertise and experience that already exists within your committee members. Remember, though, to take into consideration the amount of time your individual committee members are willing and able to dedicate to the formation of the HIE.

When you understand the skill sets, expertise required, and the level of commitments your stakeholders are willing and able to make, you can then identify where you have gaps. Then you can use outside resources to fill those gaps.

Assessing Outside Resources

There are several specific criteria you need to consider when you engage a consulting firm. Any firm that you consider engaging must have a solid history of performance in healthcare and in HIE. Many consulting firms have solid formation expertise in other industries. However, you need a firm with solid HIE formation experience. Make sure that you engage only those firms that can demonstrate hands-on experience in HIE. Ensure that they have actually done the work that they claim to have done with HIE.

In addition to ensuring that potential firms have experience in HIE, you must also ensure that they are capable of assigning resources with appropriate and demonstrated experience to your project. It is not enough that the firm has experience. You want experienced *people* on your project.

Make sure you have these experienced consultants actively working with you on a regular basis. Ensure that the people you interview from the firm are the ones who will be assigned to your project. Some firms have been known to present their highly credentialed people during the sales process in order to convince you to engage them, but when the project starts, the firm sends in their junior staff people who do not have the credentials or experience in HIE that you need. Those impressive people with the great credentials that you met in the interview process are now nowhere to be found, or they are said to be in the background "monitoring the project."

Another key component that you should insist on in a consultant, at least in the early stages, is technology vendor neutrality. You need SMEs who are not partnered with, or promoting the tools of, any particular vendor. Vendor neutrality ensures that the consultants are working only in your best interests and that they are not more focused on making a sale for their technology partner than providing you with sound, objective guidance. It is too early to focus on even a technology approach at this point, let alone on a specific vendor.

Selecting Outside Resources

Once you are comfortable that a consulting firm is a good fit for your organization or project, request that they submit a proposal. It is not always necessary to go through a formal request for proposal (RFP) process—especially if you are not a public entity—but it is always important to obtain a proposal from the firm you are considering. Use the proposal as a discussion document and as a basis of agreement for the work that you need them to perform and the fees they will charge. Ideally, developing the proposal should be a collaborative process between you and the consulting firm. The resulting proposal should designate the specific persons who will be assigned to your project.

Make sure you request references for the firm and the proposed consultants. The references should be from organizations for which the firm and individual consultants have done work that specifically relates to HIEs. Check those references! We have seen times in which a consultant's claims in their proposal were overstated or even false. In many cases, those claims were accepted without verification—to the eventual detriment of the client organization.

Choosing outside firms to help with your HIE formation can be a daunting task. Involve someone with experience in procuring outside resources. This expertise may reside within your Steering Committee or in a stakeholder organization that offers to assist you at no cost to you. Ensure that there are enough people involved in the decision making so that you can be sure that you have selected a consulting firm based upon your organization's needs and the credentials, experience, and expertise of the consultant—not solely on someone's individual preferences. For steps on the process of selecting the right SME or consulting firm for your efforts, see Figure 3-12.

CHAPTER SUMMARY

In this chapter, we have covered forming your Steering Committee and developing your organization's Vision and Mission Statements. We have also discussed how obtaining letters of commitment from your stakeholders can solidify their involvement and demonstrate to the community that this is a viable effort. These commitment letters can also be used as a step in obtaining your early funding.

We discussed using fundraising efforts of non-profit organizations within your own community as examples of how you might pursue your own fundraising.

Finally, we discussed bringing in outside expertise to help fill gaps in the expertise you will need to form an HIE. In this discussion, we took you through the steps of engaging a consulting firm and cautioned you on how to ensure that you retain the most qualified firm—and consultants—to work with you.

Upon completion of the work in this chapter, you will have:
- A functioning Steering Committee;
- Organization Vision and Mission Statements;
- Signed letters of commitment;
- A plan for obtaining early funding;

> ❏ 1. Understand what expertise you need to secure from the subject matter expert (SME) or SMEs.
>
> ❏ 2. Identify consulting firms that have specific experience and expertise in HIE formation.
>
> ❏ 3. Develop your selection criteria.
>
> ❏ 4. Through reference checks and due diligence, ensure that any individuals or consulting firms you are considering have the experience, knowledge, and appropriate personality fit to work with your developing HIE.
>
> ❏ 5. Request a proposal from the firm that describes the work they will perform and the fees they will charge.
>
> ❏ 6. Carefully check references on the consultant(s) you are considering.
>
> ❏ 7. Review final reports from candidates' past work, if possible.
>
> ❏ 8. Choose firm.
>
> ❏ 9. Negotiate contract.

Figure 3-12: Checklist—Choosing the Right SME or Consulting Firm

- An approach to procuring any required outside subject matter expertise; and
- Continued to incorporate stakeholder engagement into all of your plans and activities.

In the next chapter, we discuss how you develop your governance and transition into a more formal organization. Assuming you have followed the steps in this chapter, you are well prepared for the next step.

RESOURCES

See Appendix A for examples of Vision and Mission Statements from operating HIEs.

Grossman JM, Kushner KL, November EA. Creating Sustainable Local Health Information Exchanges: Can Barriers to Stakeholder Participation Be Overcome? Posted February 2008. http://www.hschange.org/CONTENT/970/. Accessed September, 2010.

American Planning Association. Choosing a Consultant. http://www.planning.org/consultants/choosing/. Accessed September, 2010.

Washburn S, Scanlan J, Shays EM. How to Hire a Management Consultant (Government Edition). 2006. http://www.imcusa.org/resource/resmgr/files/h2h_2008_government_version.pdf. Accessed September, 2010.

Department of Health & Human Services, Health Information Technology. (This website is a wonderful resource with the most current publicly available information about a variety of health IT related programs and topics.) http://healthit.hhs.gov/portal/server.pt?open=512&objID=1204&parentname=CommunityPage&parentid=1&mode=2&in_hi_userid=10741&cached=true. Accessed September, 2010.

Pennsylvania eHealth Initiative (PAeHI). Overview: Pennsylvania eHealth Initiative, Mission Statement and Purpose Statement. http://www.paehi.org/ehealth/overview/. Accessed September, 2010.

CHAPTER 4

Establish a Formal Organizational Governance Structure

Governance is the means by which you ensure that the organization's policies, processes, and procedures are appropriate, implemented correctly, and effective.

INTRODUCTION

A sustainable HIE requires, and depends upon, the trust of its participants. Good governance plays a key role in efforts to engage stakeholders and promote their continued interest and participation. Here we briefly discuss the relationship of good governance to continued stakeholder engagement.

"Governance is underappreciated."
Dick Thompson, Executive Director/CEO, Quality Health Network

Over time, your stakeholders will tell you what they consider to be appropriate governance. In earlier chapters, we discussed the need for engaging your stakeholders early and often and encouraging two-way communication. By understanding what your stakeholders value—what concerns them—and incorporating their input into your policies and procedures, you will be able to form the type of governance structure that supports your success and sustainability.

At some point, as you move forward in forming your HIE, you need to establish a formal governance structure for the organization. It is important to establish this organizational structure to provide the necessary framework for defining the roles and responsibilities, financial management and accountability, business operations, and oversight that will be used for running your HIE organization.

There are many activities involved in developing a formal governance structure for your organization. In Chapter 3, *Navigating Your Early Stage Formation*, we discussed one of the first steps, creating your Vision and Mission Statements. As you move forward in developing your governance structure, you need to frequently revisit your Vision and Mission Statements. It is important that you remain familiar with these statements because they form the foundation on which your organization will be built and will guide you throughout its development and operation. You will also use the results of your initial community assessment (see Chapter 2, *Getting Started*) and additional knowledge about your stakeholders (see Chapter 3, *Navigating Your Early Stage Formation*) to inform the type of governance model that will be best suited for your community.

In this chapter, we discuss the responsibilities of a formal Board of Directors and some of the key policies you need to put in place to ensure accountability and legal compliance. Because many of the policies you develop will govern your organization's privacy practices, you should become very familiar with the contents of Chapter 7, *Protecting Patient Privacy*, as you address those related policies.

In some cases, the organization that began as the HIE's "incubator" (the organization with fiduciary accountability) may stay on as the parent organization. More often, however, the HIE in its early formative stage is only temporarily housed by another organization and is then set up as a separate legal entity as soon as it is feasible. The timing of this will vary depending upon your specific circumstances.

ATTRIBUTES OF GOOD GOVERNANCE

Good governance is the organizational glue that keeps your stakeholders participating. In Chapter 6, *Your Business Plan Defines How Delivering Value Drives Your Sustainability*, we discuss various financial models that you may want to consider as you move forward; however, even the best financial model in the world is not sustainable without good governance. How do you know what kind of governance is right for your HIE? Your stakeholders will tell you. Ask them. Examples of the attributes of good governance are found in the governance attributes in the State HIE Cooperative Agreement Program Grant RFP.[1] These are summarized in Figure 4-1.

CRITERIA FOR GOOD HIE GOVERNANCE

Good HIE governance models meet four basic criteria. A good HIE governance model is:

- Able to promote trust in the HIE within your community;
- Consistent with the norms of your community;
- Consistent with the organization's current stage of development or operation; and
- Adaptable to changes in the environment.

Promotes Trust within Your Community

Good governance is critical to maintaining trust in your organization. The governance model you choose, and the way you conduct business, needs to be open and transparent. This means that you are sensitive to the needs of your stakeholders to be actively involved in governance and that they feel secure in how your HIE operates.

Consistent with the Norms of Your Community

The governance model that you adopt needs to be consistent with the norms of your community. There are different levels of need for decision making, control, and transparency in different communities. You must be sensitive to, and respect, your community norms.

1. Establish a governance structure that achieves broad-based stakeholder collaboration with transparency, buy-in, and trust.

2. Set goals, objectives, and performance measures for the exchange of health information that reflect consensus among the healthcare stakeholder groups and that accomplish coverage of all providers for HIE requirements related to meaningful use criteria to be established by the Secretary [of HHS] through the rule-making process.

3. Ensure the coordination, integration, and alignment of efforts with Medicaid and public health programs through efforts of the State Health IT Coordinators.

4. Establish mechanisms to provide oversight and accountability of HIE to protect the public interest.

5. Account for the flexibility needed to align with emerging nationwide HIE governance that will be specified in future program guidance.

Figure 4-1: Governance Attributes Found in the State HIE Cooperative Agreement Program Grant RFP. (Adapted from the Department of Health & Human Services, Office of the National Coordinator for Health Information Technology. State Health Information Exchange Cooperative Agreement Program, Funding Opportunity Announcement. 2009; 15.)

Consistent with the Organization's Current Stage of Development or Operation

The governance model that you create must be consistent with the current stage of your development. Are you just beginning? Are you in the early formation stage at which your needs may be informal? On the other hand, are you moving into operations where you are going to be managing finances and other resources? These factors influence the selection—and appropriateness of—your governance model.

Adaptable to Changes in the Environment

Good HIE governance needs to be able to adapt to the changing healthcare environment. You must be able to adjust as new rules, regulations, and laws are put into place. This has implications for how you write your bylaws, how specific or general your policies are, and how you develop and modify your organization's processes and procedures.

DEVELOP ORGANIZATIONAL PRINCIPLES

Principles describe what you value as an organization. Organizational principles are statements that describe the manner in which an organization goes about its business. They are statements that describe your organization's beliefs and its intended behavior when it interacts with your stakeholders and the community. Principles should be positively worded and aspirational. Figure 4-2 provides examples of some of the organizational governance principles that we have gathered through our work with various HIEs.

1. Patients come first.

2. The board, and its individual members, always act in the best interest of the community we serve.

3. Consumer privacy, security, and confidentiality are paramount.

4. Multi-stakeholder collaboration is needed to implement achievable and measureable initiatives.

5. Senior leadership on the governing body is necessary for the HIE initiative to accomplish its goals.

6. Governing body composition should be sized to get work done and include all critical stakeholder interests.

7. Governing body composition must have balanced stakeholder representation.

8. The governing body should make appointments to workgroups based on the skills and competencies needed to carry out the work.

9. Rules of engagement for interacting and communicating with stakeholders must be set early and administered consistently.

10. The formative governing body (steering committee or early board) must commit to putting in the required time—and staying in place—until the formative work is done.

11. The processes for governing body development and selection, as well as participation in other volunteer roles, must be explicit and transparent.

12. Bylaws and other establishing documents should be designed to allow reasonable flexibility, to the extent permitted by law, so the organization may adapt as early lessons are learned.

13. HIE governing bodies must follow all established practices for legal and effective governance.

14. It is imperative that the governing body members serve the interest of the HIE by thinking above their own organizations' immediate interests and holding to the vision and the long-term goal of healthcare data sharing.

15. The needs of the organization will likely change over time, and the governing body may need to undergo a series of transitions to remain effective.

Figure 4-2: Examples of HIE Organizational Governance Principles

According to Trudi Matthews, HealthBridge, a major reason their stakeholders trust them is because of their principles. She stresses the importance of, early on, establishing clear guiding principles for your organization. An example she provided of a key guiding principle for HealthBridge is to *never* share confidential business information with or among the participants (such as which physicians are prescribing what drugs or which providers are using specific hospitals). Other principles critical to their success are to focus on data sharing for treatment purposes and never to sell clinical information.

THE BOARD OF DIRECTORS

The specific make up and responsibilities of a Board of Directors may vary across organizations. However, there are general accountabilities that are common across most boards. The following are some of those accountabilities:

- Setting overall direction for the organization;
- Setting and maintaining fiduciary accountability for the organization;
- Setting expectations for the community being served and being accountable to the community for meeting those expectations;
- Approving the budget;
- Developing the organization's strategy to accomplish its objectives;
- Accepting or rejecting recommendations from Advisory Groups; and
- Holding the executive director (or CEO) accountable for performance of the organization.

Leading practices show that a team consisting of somewhere between six and eight individuals is the ideal size for effective decision making. This is big enough to represent a diverse range of opinions but still small enough to get to a decision. The size of your board will depend heavily upon the roles you choose for the members and your HIE's overall decision-making approach.

Laura Adams, President & CEO of the Rhode Island Quality Institute, pointed out that "[HIE] boards are unlike any traditional non-profit board. This board is part and parcel of your organization. Unlike other boards with "outsiders," this is vastly different. They are the (only) people who can make change happen. They are the conduit by which any transformation is accomplished. You have to be prepared to tolerate and genuinely appreciate much deeper engagement by the board than you would experience with other organizations."

The following are some characteristics of well-functioning boards:

- Highly competent members
- Well-coordinated
- Collegial
- Focused on unambiguous goals

The board will evolve over time as it adjusts to environmental changes and the maturation of the organization. Stakeholder levels of interest and active participation will change as the organization evolves, so it is only logical that the makeup of your board may change as well. While you may be required by statute or bylaws to have some permanent board seats, you should continue to ensure that your board represents a diverse set of stakeholder perspectives.

In large boards, an Executive Committee usually meets more frequently than the entire board. They may make certain decisions (within the bylaws) or put together for the board an agenda consisting of their recommendations.

> Examine the
> governance models
> of other successful
> community-based
> organizations in
> your community.

Consensus is an important component of the success of HIE efforts. We recommend that the Executive Committee be the group that conducts in-depth inquiries into, and fully discusses, those issues that are considered board-level issues. They can then provide the background of the issue, present their research, and recommend a course of action to the board. The board then has the opportunity to further discuss and understand those recommendations, modify them as needed, and then to reach consensus before moving forward.

Word of caution: With the consensus approach, there is always the possibility of someone attempting to block a decision or block forward progress on an issue. If this happens, remind the individual of your basic principles—one of these should be that the board and its members are accountable to act in the *best interests of the community as a whole*—not to represent individual or specific organizational agendas.

GOVERNANCE MODELS

There are many different types of governance models. Only you and your community can determine the model that is right for your organization. We have observed that as HIEs go through the various stages of formation and operation, their governance typically evolves and matures. You may start very informally, maybe meeting at a local coffee shop over a cup of coffee, and progress to a much more formal boardroom style over time.

In the following section, we describe four common types of governance models that you may want to consider as you create your own governance. Keep in mind that what is right for you may not be the right model for other communities, and what works in other communities may not work in yours. The governance model you select may be a hybrid of the models discussed next. Understanding the different approaches can help you determine the kind of governance model you should adopt. Most importantly, you need to put in place the governance model that your stakeholders and community want and need you to have for you to be successful.

Management Team Model

This model operates according to the model of a management team and assumes the deepest level of involvement in day-to-day operations. In this model, you organize your committees and activities along functional lines. The structure of the board and its committees may mirror the organization's structure. If there is limited or no paid staff, the board's committee structure becomes the organization's de facto administrative structure and the board members actually manage and deliver the services.

The management model is often seen in organizations in the early formation stage of their development where there is a high level of board involvement in the operational and administrative duties of the organization. In the management model, decision making of the board may extend to specific details and decisions about programs, services, and administrative practices. This high level of involvement of the board should decrease as the organization matures.

Board members are selected based on their knowledge and experience in management. This model is common in start-up organizations in which staff may have specialized business, operational, or technical expertise but is limited in its general management experience.

Advisory Board Model

In this model, the board's role is primarily that of a helper or advisor to the CEO/executive director. Board members are recruited for three main reasons: they are trusted as advisers by the executive director; they have professional skills and competence that the organization needs and that it cannot or does not want to pay for; or they are likely to be helpful in establishing and demonstrating the credibility of the organization for fundraising and public relations purposes.

The drawback of an Advisory Board model is that while it can work well for a short period of time, it generally lacks the accountability mechanisms that are required of boards over the longer term. The organization, and the board, may fail to recognize that the board members can be held accountable for certain actions of the organization.

Collaborative Model

In this model, responsibility is shared and decision making is normally carried out through consensus. No individual has direct power over another. Its advocates describe this as the most democratic style of management, but it is also perhaps the most difficult of all models to maintain. Very often, the people involved may have very strong personal or professional opinions and compromise may not be their strong suit.

In the HIE, consensus building and collaboration are key critical success factors. Whatever model you select, you need to consider including at least some of the characteristics of the collaborative model—such as building consensus for decisions.

Policy Board Model

In the Policy Board model, the job of the board is to establish the guiding principles and policies for the organization and then delegate responsibility and authority to staff members who are responsible for enacting the policies. This board primarily monitors and certifies compliance.

The Policy Board model is seen most often in more mature organizations. Policy Boards are characterized by a high level of trust and confidence in the CEO or executive director. It is the job of the board to ensure that both staff, and the board itself, are held accountable for their performance. There are typically few standing committees on this type of board, and its members are recruited for their demonstrated commitment to the values and mission of the organization.

We provide examples of the different types of governance in place in various HIEs at the end of this chapter.

TESTING YOUR GOVERNANCE MODEL

Good governance is critical to your success because it solidifies the promise of trust that you make to your stakeholders. Once you decide on your governance model, you need to test it and validate that it is the right model for your organization and your community. In addition to the criteria for good governance discussed earlier, test your model on its ability to:

- Promote community trust in your organization;
- Evolve in a changing environment;
- Respond to the initial—and changing—needs of your stakeholders; and
- Include a broad cross section of your community.

Does Your Governance Model Promote Trust?

Transparency and trust are absolutes for your HIE to be successful and sustainable. One of the main purposes of governance is to make your organization reliable and predictable and, thus, trustworthy. You need to have established and clear rules, principles, and expectations. Board members need to be the type of people that your community trusts. Stakeholders, and the community at large, need to know that they can trust that their money is being spent wisely, that their privacy is being protected, and that the organization has their best interests at the forefront. Solid governance and the right board members provide the essential foundation required for that trust.

Can Your Governance Model Effectively Evolve over Time?

Why is this important? Because the needs of your organization will change over time. The environment in which you operate is constantly changing. Members of the board, and their roles, will also change over time. It seems that today, healthcare is changing faster than the speed of light. Create a governing board that can adapt to that kind and rate of change.

You may initially select board members who are influential in the community in order to help build your support and get things moving. As you evolve and become more formal, you may need to move toward a governance structure and board members who are well-suited for overseeing an ongoing operation.

Is Your Governance Able to Be Responsive to a Changing Environment?

It must be responsive to your stakeholders, to changes within your community, and to the changes in the healthcare environment in general. Are your policies able to easily accommodate external changes? As has been said frequently in the past, and now is so appropriate to our rapidly changing healthcare environment, "The only constant is that things will change."

Is Your Board Diverse and Inclusive?

Your board and your governance model need to include a broad and representative stakeholder base. Stakeholders need to feel they have been listened to and that their wants, needs, and concerns are included in the decision-making process. This is crucial to engaging them and maintaining both their initial and ongoing participation. Including your key stakeholders in your activities, and constantly communicating with them, will put you on the road to stakeholder sustainability.

Remember, even the best financial model in the world is unsustainable if the governance model does not provide the organization's stakeholders with the confidence and trust that their wants and needs—what they tell you they value—are being met. Adopt a governance model that promotes your stakeholders' continued trust in the organization.

DEVELOPING KEY POLICIES FOR YOUR ORGANIZATION

The organizational policies you develop determine the parameters and framework for the governance of the organization. They should be specific enough to be clear but not so detailed that they need to be modified for every change in your environment. Remember, the policies should reflect your core principles. Those core principles rarely change.

The following are some of the key policies and decisions you need to address as you create your organizational governance:

- Board member roles, responsibilities, and accountability
  - The type of board you will create
  - The size of the board and the makeup of its members
- How the business of the board will be conducted
- Privacy policies
- Finance policies
- Decision-making process
- Data use and reuse policies
- Operational policies

Board Roles and Responsibility

In our introduction to the Board of Directors' role earlier, we identified specific board accountabilities. Clearly defining the board's roles and responsibilities is critical to having an effective board. Here, in this section on policies, we describe in more detail some of the roles and responsibilities you will need to consider as you develop your policies. The list below provides some examples of board roles and responsibilities that you may want to include.

1. Determine or validate the organization's vision and mission.
2. Ensure effective organizational planning.
3. Govern the organization through establishing broad policies and objectives.
4. Ensure adequate resources for the organization.
5. Manage resources effectively.
6. Determine and monitor the organization's programs and services.
7. Enhance the organization's public image.
8. Assess its own performance.

Policies need to address how the board will govern and its relationship to the HIE's management, staff, and other stakeholders. Ultimately, the board is accountable to the community being served. The executive director (or CEO) is accountable to the board for the organization's operations.

Size and Makeup of the Board

Determine the number of board members and the desired, or required, qualifications of the members. This includes determining the types and amount of community representation desired on the board. Leading practices show that the board should be representative of the perspectives of all stakeholders in the community, including physicians, hospitals, ancillary services, government, payers, consumers, and other important groups in your community. Board members should also be free of conflicts of interest. It is also a leading practice to require that board members disclose any real or potential conflicts at the time they are nominated for the position.

Many boards take advantage of the wealth of expertise in the community by setting up standing advisory groups. Two common advisory groups for HIEs include a Clinical Advisory Group and a Legal Advisory Group. The members of these advisory groups generally do not actively sit on the board; instead, they are called upon as needed to provide guidance and make recommendations.

Describe How the Business of the Board Will Be Conducted

It is important to set expectations and develop policies concerning how the board itself will operate. Specify how topics will be introduced and discussed and how decisions will be made. How you run your board meetings needs to be reflective of your core principles.

For example, if transparency is a core principle, you may have policies regarding the open nature of your meetings; how the community may attend and participate; and how broadly the minutes of the meetings are distributed.

Also, consider policies relating to how the board will respond to recommendations. Is there a small Executive Committee (discussed earlier) that makes recommendations for subsequent decisions by the larger board? What is the role of advisory groups?

Policies Specific to Protecting Patient Privacy

The board will work closely with the Privacy workgroup to develop the appropriate polices that relate to protecting patient privacy. Some examples of the policies that the board must address are those relating to:

- Patient consent—Opt in, opt-out, or no opt. Many states are now addressing this on a statewide basis, and you need to know where your state stands. The ONC issued a report in March, 2010 on "Consumer Consent Options for Electronic HIE: Policy Considerations and Analysis"[2] that provides an excellent reference as you formulate your policies in this area. Also, the Tiger Team,[3] formed by ONC in June, 2010, is in the process developing consent-related policies as this book is being written.
- Data Use and Reciprocal Services Agreements (DURSA)[4]—These are trust agreements that are used by the Nationwide Health Information Network (NHIN) participants to provide mutual assurance of data privacy.
- Business Associate Agreements (BAAs)—These were first required under HIPAA for organizations sharing patient information. ARRA has expanded the number and types of entities that now must participate in BAAs to include,

among others, health information exchange organizations. Please refer to the references at the end of this chapter for resources containing a more in-depth discussion of BAAs.

- Accountability—Accountability and punishment for intentional data security breaches.

A more in-depth discussion of privacy and the policies necessary to conform to current laws and regulations can be found in Chapter 7, *Protecting Patient Privacy*.

Finance Policies

The board will work closely with the Business & Finance workgroup to develop the key policies relating to the handling of finances. You need to ensure that you comply with all relevant federal, state, and local regulations.

Other Key Policies

In addition to the policy areas just discussed, there are additional policies you need to consider. Some of these address the following questions:

- How will you handle publicity and talking with the media in the event you have "bad news" to deliver?
- What are your human resources and staffing policies? You need to comply with all relevant federal and state laws.
- How will you handle potential strategic investments?
- What will happen in the event of a "change of control" for your organization, e.g., if you should merge with another organization?

Each of your policies must also be supplemented with associated procedures. The procedures should describe *how* your organization will implement each policy.

CREATING YOUR BYLAWS

No matter what type of organization you decide to form, you most likely will need bylaws to show the state how you intend to operate. At the end of this chapter, we provide resources and links to some good examples of bylaws in use by operating HIEs. Many of these organizations are readily willing to share their bylaws with other HIE efforts.

Use the checklist in Figure 4-3 as a tool to remind you of the key points and activities involved in forming your organizational governance.

FORMING A LEGAL ENTITY—IF APPROPRIATE

If you do choose to become a separate legal entity, there are some specific activities you need to complete to fulfill the legal requirements of becoming an independent organization. We recommend that you seek legal counsel as you grapple with the laws specific to your state and region.

The Most Common Type of Legal Entity for HIE

There are many types of legal entities under which a business may decide to formally organize. There are for-profit entities and not-for-profit entities. By far, the most common legal entity for the HIE is the not-for-profit. By forming a not-for-profit entity, you

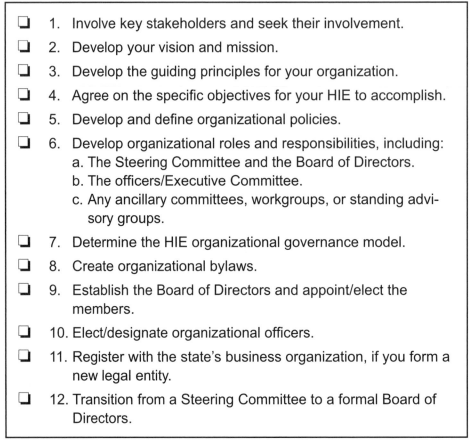

❏   1. Involve key stakeholders and seek their involvement.

❏   2. Develop your vision and mission.

❏   3. Develop the guiding principles for your organization.

❏   4. Agree on the specific objectives for your HIE to accomplish.

❏   5. Develop and define organizational policies.

❏   6. Develop organizational roles and responsibilities, including:
       a. The Steering Committee and the Board of Directors.
       b. The officers/Executive Committee.
       c. Any ancillary committees, workgroups, or standing advi-
          sory groups.

❏   7. Determine the HIE organizational governance model.

❏   8. Create organizational bylaws.

❏   9. Establish the Board of Directors and appoint/elect the
       members.

❏   10. Elect/designate organizational officers.

❏   11. Register with the state's business organization, if you form a
        new legal entity.

❏   12. Transition from a Steering Committee to a formal Board of
        Directors.

Figure 4-3: Checklist—Creating Formal Organizational Governance

can investigate if you may be eligible to apply to become a 501(c)3 organization under the U.S. Internal Revenue Service (IRS) regulations. Attaining 501(c)3 status will enable you to apply for a wide variety of government and other grants and may also provide those who donate to your organization the possibility of claiming the donation as a charitable contribution. To attain 501(c)3 status you will need the explicit approval of the IRS. In the past, obtaining this approval was a slow and arduous process as the IRS sought to fully understand the concept of an HIE organization. However, it seems that recently more HIE organizations have been receiving approval of their 501(c)3 status. Make sure you seek solid legal counsel as you determine the type of legal entity and tax designation status that is right for your organization.

Figure 4-4 lists some of the high-level steps that you need to include if you decide to pursue becoming an independent legal entity.

THE EXECUTIVE DIRECTOR

In this book, we refer to the lead staff position in the HIE as the executive director. Others may call it the chief executive officer (CEO), president, or some other title. The executive director is the person who will not only provide another resource for community outreach, but will become the person that the community identifies as the face of the HIE. It is important to have a full-time position dedicated to coordinating activi-

---

❏ 1. Determine the appropriate type of legal entity for your organization:
   a. For-profit or not-for-profit
   b. Corporation
   c. LLC, etc.

❏ 2. Determine the name of your organization, and ensure that it is available.

❏ 3. Write and approve your bylaws.

❏ 4. Create and approve your articles of incorporation.

❏ 5. Determine who you will list as the responsible parties for the organization on your business application.

❏ 6. Complete all of the activities required to register as a legal entity in your state, county, and city.

❏ 7. Obtain business license(s) as required.

❏ 8. Acquire a Federal Employer Identification Number (FEIN).

❏ 9. File for a DUNS number. The Data Universal Numbering System, abbreviated as DUNS or D-U-N-S, is a system developed and regulated by Dun & Bradstreet (D&B) that assigns a unique numeric identifier, referred to as a DUNS number, to a single business entity.

❏ 10. Obtain board liability insurance.

❏ 11. Establish your finance and accounting procedures.

❏ 12. Apply for appropriate tax status, if needed.

Figure 4-4: Checklist—Becoming a Legal Entity

ties early in the development of your HIE. The executive director may be hired at any time during the course of the formation of the HIE—typically once there is a consistent source of funding; however, it is essential to bring someone into this position as early as possible. In some cases, this might be a volunteer, but be aware that this should be a full-time, paid position. Regardless of his or her employment status with the HIE, the person should have strong motivation and the skills to build a solid organization. Look for someone who is experienced in successfully building an organization or business. The right person in this position is critical to your success. As Laura Adams, of the Rhode Island Quality Institute states, "[You] need the most talented strategic person that you can engage. Get people who are comfortable with leading amid ambiguity and who won't make small-minded mistakes."

Executive Director Roles, Responsibilities, and Accountability

The executive director is accountable to the board for the overall performance of the organization. As such, this person must be given the appropriate level of authority and resources to carry out that responsibility. Typically, the executive director is an ex-officio (non-voting) member of the board. In a good executive director/board relationship, both realize that the executive director's accountability is not an assignment from the board but is a mutual transaction in which the executive director successfully manages the organization and the board provides the environment and the resources to promote that success.

In some cases, organizations have initially tried to get by solely with volunteers, only to discover that there are too many responsibilities and activities to handle and coordinate on a part-time or volunteer basis. A leading practice for successful HIE efforts is to invest resources early in a full-time position—bringing in someone who can represent the organization, coordinate the activities and drive the execution of the mission. In other words, this person is accountable for the successful formation and operation of the HIE.

The following are examples of executive director accountabilities:
- Build the organization
- Manage finances
- Manage the organization's performance
- Hire and manage staff
- Make contractual agreements
- Provide training

Initially a full-time, interim project manager with outreach responsibilities may be considered. If there is a strong management-focused board with time to commit to the effort, the forming HIE may be able to defer the hiring of an executive director. However, we do not recommend that you delay in hiring someone to fill this critical position.

Hiring the Executive Director

Before you seek candidates for the position, you must have a clear idea of what responsibilities and accountabilities this position encompasses. You also need to identify the skills and competencies any candidate needs in order to fulfill the role. Write a job description for the position, which clearly delineates the incumbent's role and authority. The board should approve the job description.

Consider securing help and advice from someone with experience in creating job descriptions, preferably someone who also has experience in describing job roles and responsibilities for leading an organization. You may want to hire a professional search firm to locate candidates for the position or you may decide to hire a consultant or contractor as an interim executive director. In either case, consider seeking advice to ensure that your hiring criteria, compensation plans, and other benefits are within the laws and norms for your community and will meet your HIE's needs.

The hiring decision should be a consensus decision by the board since the person brought in will have to work collaboratively with all board members. This means that the board members should be actively involved in the interview and selection process. Once a candidate is selected, the board chair should make the offer of employment to, or negotiate a contract with, that person. A summary of the steps involved in hiring an executive director is shown in Figure 4-5.

❑ 1. Define roles and responsibility for the position.

❑ 2. Develop accountability description.

❑ 3. Create job description.

❑ 4. Approve job description.

❑ 5. Determine compensation and other employment terms.

❑ 6. Develop criteria for ideal candidate.

❑ 7. Search for applicants.

❑ 8. Review and evaluate applications.

❑ 9. Have several board members interview job applicants.

❑ 10. Board members responsible for making the hiring decision discuss the various candidates.

❑ 11. Get consensus on the successful candidate.

❑ 12. Chair of board or designate make the job offer.

❑ 13. Negotiate and agree on employment contract.

❑ 14. Selected candidate signs employment contract.

Figure 4-5: Checklist—Hiring the Executive Director

CREATING WORKGROUPS

In the formation phase, there is a lot of work to do, and it involves all five of the HIE activity and competency domains that we introduced in Chapter 2, *Getting Started*, and Chapter 3, *Navigating Your Early Stage Formation*. Our experience shows that an effective way to approach this is through forming five workgroups—each focused on one of the HIE domains. The workgroups should be comprised of members who have specific domain knowledge and expertise. As you move through the formation phase, there will be times that the individual workgroups need to work together, on an ad hoc basis, to address cross-domain issues. At other times, the work of one group may be dependent upon the completion of certain activities by another workgroup. This is typical behavior for large, complex projects. At the risk of repeating ourselves, forming an HIE is a large, complex change management project.

The key to successfully managing all of these efforts is having solid communication across and among these workgroups and a strong central management team that keeps the workgroups focused and on track. This generally is the responsibility of the executive director.

In your HIE formation, we recommend that the inclusion of the clinical perspective be an integral part of each of the workgroups. After all, if the output of the group does not meet the needs of your clinical stakeholders, your chances for success are severely limited.

As mentioned in Chapter 3, *Navigating Your Early Stage Formation*, the workgroups you should consider forming are:

- Stakeholder Engagement & Participation
- Governance
- Business & Finance
- Privacy
- Technology & Security

The workgroup members will not necessarily be board members, but each workgroup should include at least one board member—who may also lead the workgroup. As with your board members, you may want to consider requiring members of your workgroups to also declare any real or potential conflicts of interest.

In addition to forming these workgroups, you need to identify subject matter experts (SMEs) in the legal, clinical, and health information exchange fields who can act as advisors to the groups.

Primary Workgroups and Their Purpose

HIE workgroup success depends upon having, and adhering to, a clearly defined purpose with associated objectives. It also depends upon developing a good roadmap and effectively implementing the work plan. Charters are a tool that workgroups can use to help ensure their success. A charter is an agreement among workgroup members outlining how the team will work together, make decisions, and share accountability for delivering high-quality work products. A charter is especially important in volunteer HIE workgroups because members often come from organizations with different styles of management, decision making, accountability, communication, and levels of business acumen. The success of each domain workgroup rests on the shared understanding and mutual commitment to a set of principles and practices that describe how the domain team will work together and achieve its objectives.

Developing a workgroup charter involves more than just filling out a template and having each workgroup member sign it. The ability of the charter to effectively guide a team depends on the process by which it is developed and the negotiated accountabilities and authorities embedded in the charter document. Each charter is unique, depending on the required tasks, the skills and capabilities of its members, and the constraints under which the workgroup operates. This means you need to clearly specify the desired capabilities of the workgroup members, their roles, agreed-upon work processes, their specific work products and deliverables, and their relationships to other workgroups. These "rules of operation" are contained in the workgroup charter.

A workgroup charter cannot just be signed and then filed away. The charter is a living document, representing the workgroup's operating principles and should be referred to frequently. Depending on how the work of the group proceeds, it may even be necessary to modify the charter to accommodate unforeseen or emerging conditions or circumstances.

Finally, it is useful to designate a single individual to serve as facilitator and advisor to workgroups for charter development. An "HIE charter facilitator" (who could be an existing Executive Team member or an independent consultant) could accelerate the charter development and approval process and promote consistency across all workgroups. This consistency is important because it promotes coordination among workgroups through the HIE formation process.

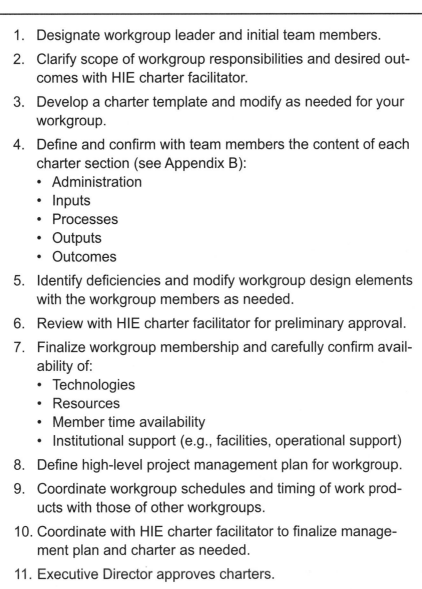

❏　1.　Designate workgroup leader and initial team members.

❏　2.　Clarify scope of workgroup responsibilities and desired outcomes with HIE charter facilitator.

❏　3.　Develop a charter template and modify as needed for your workgroup.

❏　4.　Define and confirm with team members the content of each charter section (see Appendix B):
• Administration
• Inputs
• Processes
• Outputs
• Outcomes

❏　5.　Identify deficiencies and modify workgroup design elements with the workgroup members as needed.

❏　6.　Review with HIE charter facilitator for preliminary approval.

❏　7.　Finalize workgroup membership and carefully confirm availability of:
• Technologies
• Resources
• Member time availability
• Institutional support (e.g., facilities, operational support)

❏　8.　Define high-level project management plan for workgroup.

❏　9.　Coordinate workgroup schedules and timing of work products with those of other workgroups.

❏　10.　Coordinate with HIE charter facilitator to finalize management plan and charter as needed.

❏　11.　Executive Director approves charters.

❏　12.　Execute charter by members signing the final charter.

Figure 4-6: Checklist—Developing Workgroup Charters

Creating a Workgroup Charter

We recommend the steps shown in Figure 4-6 to help you develop a charter for each of your workgroups. Additional details and examples of charter contents can be found in Appendix B.

Although optional, a high-level charter for the HIE formation project is advisable. However, before any workgroup finalizes its charter and begins its activities, it should review at least a preliminary version of the charters for each of the other domains. Moving ahead with one domain before the cross workgroup coordination design and processes are in place often leads to rework and delays.

Next, we provide brief sample descriptions of the responsibilities of each workgroup.

Stakeholder Engagement & Participation Workgroup

The Stakeholder Engagement & Participation workgroup will drive the organization's activities to involve stakeholders and maintain their engagement in the HIE. This group is also responsible for developing and driving the implementation of the communication plan. They are responsible for identifying ways to participate in community events at which the HIE can be highlighted; obtaining stakeholder input required by other workgroups; and developing the overall approach for engaging stakeholders and keeping them interested and participating in the HIE. Each of the other workgroups should regularly coordinate and work with this group to ensure that they are including adequate stakeholder input, feedback, and buy-in as they develop their own recommendations. In addition, this group, by understanding the activities being undertaken by the other groups, should proactively identify opportunities for communicating and discussing the HIE's mission, objectives, and accomplishments with the community as a whole.

Governance Workgroup

The Governance workgroup will drive the formation of the legal and governing structures of the HIE. This group will define expectations, policies, roles, and responsibilities, decision-making approaches, and accountability. They work closely with the Privacy workgroup as the privacy policies are developed.

Business & Finance Workgroup

The Business & Finance workgroup will lead the development of the strategic and business plans for the HIE. This group defines the business model and creates the revenue plan. Stakeholder engagement and participation are key to the success of this group. They will coordinate with the Stakeholder Engagement & Participation workgroup to ensure that they have an appropriate understanding of stakeholder wants and needs by monitoring focus groups, conducting surveys, and by obtaining feedback on the service offerings they propose, develop, and implement. This group is also responsible for recommending the initial HIE budget and developing the participation agreements.

Privacy Workgroup

The Privacy workgroup will develop the policies and procedures that are necessary to protect a patient's health information. This group is responsible for ensuring that the privacy policies meet all applicable state and federal regulations. A solid understanding of the legal ramifications of privacy is a critical foundation for the members of this group. In addition, the members need a good understanding of the current work at the federal and state levels in this area. This group should include someone with legal expertise in the field of HIE privacy. Also, since the security policies will support the privacy policies, this group should work closely with the security experts on the Technology & Security workgroup.

Technology & Security Workgroup

The Technology & Security workgroup will design the overall technical architecture for the HIE, design the physical and technical security approaches, recommend the technology service model, evaluate vendor solutions, and recommend a technology vendor. Early on, the Business & Finance workgroup will need some high-level estimates of the costs associated with technology as they begin their budgeting process. This group will provide those estimates but with the caveat that the estimate they provide most likely will change drastically as the technology approach is further defined and a specific technology implementation path is chosen.

DIRECTING AND MANAGING THE VARIOUS WORKGROUPS

The initial tasks of each workgroup are to understand their charter, recommend refinements, and gain the board's approval to move forward. A qualified workgroup leader should also be identified. As we indicated earlier, the leader may be a sitting member of the board.

The leader of each workgroup is responsible for driving the group to complete their responsibilities. This person will report the progress of the group to the appropriate management structure overseeing the workgroup activities and work with other workgroup leaders to ensure that each group's work is aligned with that of the other groups.

An active, formal project management approach should be employed at this point. The work (and outputs) of each workgroup is complex and coordinating the groups requires a structured approach to ensure the effort is well-managed. Consider contracting with a project manager who is experienced in managing diverse projects with a significant technical component.

Figure 4-7 provides a high-level checklist for the activities needed to create, launch, and manage these workgroups.

❏ 1. Develop initial charters for each of the workgroups.

❏ 2. Identify candidates who possess the desired skill sets for membership in the workgroups.

❏ 3. Recruit selected candidates to serve on a voluntary basis.

❏ 4. Identify a leader for each group who will have the responsibility to drive the workgroup to completion of their assigned tasks and who also reports progress made to the appropriate board level oversight body.

❏ 5. Formally launch each workgroup.

❏ 6. Actively manage the workgroups as part of an overall project management plan.

❏ 7. As the outputs from the workgroups are delivered, integrate them into your overall plans.

Figure 4-7: Checklist—Creating and Managing Workgroups

- Vision and mission are approved.
- The organization's basic principles have been created and adopted.
- Formal governance policies and procedures are adopted.
- Initial board roles and responsibilities are documented.
- Bylaws are adopted.
- A formal Board of Directors has been appointed or elected.
- Officers/executive committee are identified.
- Articles of incorporation are filed.

Figure 4-8: Key Components of a Formal Governance Structure

ORGANIZATIONAL COMPONENTS IN PLACE WHEN GOVERNANCE IS FORMED

Your initial work in developing the formal organizational structure will be complete when you have created and adopted the components listed in Figure 4-8. These are the key components of a formal governance structure. While your governance structure will continue to mature and evolve over time, these components ensure that your governance is built on a solid foundation.

WHY THIS IS JUST THE BEGINNING

This is just the beginning of the work for your Board of Directors. The board is the designated body accountable for ensuring that the workgroups are well coordinated, aligned to the mission and principles of your organization, and that they deliver on their charters. The Board members have now assumed formal responsibility for promoting the mission of the organization, and their responsibilities include legal and fiduciary accountability for the organization. The roles and activities of your governance structure will evolve over time as your organization matures through the formation stage into the operational stage.

CHAPTER SUMMARY

In this chapter, we have addressed the overall components, attributes, and principles of good HIE governance. The role of the board was discussed. We reviewed several potential governance models for you to consider and discussed several of the policies that you should put in place to govern the organization.

We addressed the steps needed to form an independent legal entity and also the hiring of the executive director. We also discussed the workgroups that will be involved in developing the various components necessary to form an HIE. Lastly, we highlighted the need to adopt a formal project management approach to coordinate and monitor the activities of the workgroups.

When you complete the work in this chapter, you will have:

- Chosen the appropriate initial members for your Board of Directors.
- Developed your organizational principles.

- Created a Board of Directors that operates according to your principles and in accordance with the attributes of good governance.
- A basic understanding of the work to be done to develop your organizational policies.
- An understanding of the high-level steps to becoming an independent legal entity.
- Hired your executive director.
- Launched the five workgroups that together will undertake and complete the work necessary to form the HIE.

CASE STUDIES

Delaware Health Information Network (DHIN)

Gina Bianco Perez, Executive Director, Delaware Health Information Network

According to Gina Perez, DHIN's governance consists of a public-private partnership. The private sector includes stakeholders from consumers, hospitals, labs, health plans, and multiple doctors' practices. The public sector includes the state of Delaware government, DHSS, the Department of Insurance, the Office of Technology and Information, and the Office of Management and Budget.

The Board of Directors, which meets quarterly, is made up of 60% private sector individuals. The Executive Committee, which meets twice a month, is made up of representatives from each stakeholder group. There are also the following committees that drive operations:

- Project Management
- Consumer Advisory
- Clinical Advisory
- HIM (Health Information Management)
- Finance
- Transitions of Care Workgroup

The state legislation set up how board members are appointed, the voting rules, and board responsibilities. Decisions require a quorum of the organizations represented. Committees make recommendations and the board may make additional suggestions or vote to approve the committee recommendations

According to Perez, keeping stakeholders participating is critical to the success of an HIE. She recommends conducting meaningful meetings that anyone interested is welcome to attend.

HealthInfoNet

Devore Culver, Executive Director and CEO, HealthInfoNet

HealthInfoNet in Maine is a 501(c)3 not-for-profit organization. They have a community board, which currently has 21 members who were chosen because of who they are, not by the organizations that they represent. Their bylaws, which can be found at http://www.hinfonet.org/docs/ByLaws.pdf, specify:

- Stakeholder responsibility
- Minimum number of participating members

- The three public members appointed by the governor
- Categories of representation

There are two standing committees:

- Technical and Professional Advisory Committee
- Consumer Advisory Committee

All members of the board vote, and board decisions are made by majority. The exception to this is that decisions to change the bylaws require a two-thirds majority for approval.

HealthBridge

Trudi Matthews, Director of Policy and Public Relations, HealthBridge

Headquartered in Cincinnati, Ohio, HealthBridge has a multi-stakeholder board comprising 12 members. It consists of representatives from employers, public health, health plans, and community organizations—including local, physician, and hospital associations—as well as individual hospitals and physicians. The initial organizational subscribers still hold board seats, and that group consists of four hospitals and two health plans.

Decisions are frequently made by consensus; however, each seat gets one vote.

Arizona Health-e Connection (AzHeC)

Brad Tritle, Executive Director, Arizona Health-e Connection

Arizona Health-e Connection (AzHeC) is a 501(c)3 non-profit organization with a Board of Directors (limited to 25 members), an Executive Committee, and multiple additional committees. Seven board members are permanent members and the remaining non-permanent members are elected on an annual basis. The permanent members consist of institutions that are from the state or statewide, including the Governor's Office, Medicaid, Department of Health, Arizona State CIO, Arizona Medical Association, Osteopathic Association, and Arizona Hospital and Healthcare Association.

The remaining seats are held by the following representative categories of stakeholders:

- Up to five health plans
- One lab
- One pharmacy or pharmacy association
- Two hospitals
- Up to five Medical Trading Area representatives, including a Tribal/Indian healthcare representative
- Up to three at-large members; currently, these members represent Telemedicine, Medicare QIO, and Consumers
- Higher education
- Two employer or employer association representatives

Cooperation and leadership skills among the members are important to successful operation. AzHeC seeks individuals who can get an issue worked through to resolution and consensus by using his or her leadership skills to help the group collaborate to reach solutions. Everyone on the board has a single vote; however, key decisions are made by consensus.

There are also approximately ten organizational members annually from outside the board that pay to be members of the organization, and these members elect the board. Other member categories such as vendor supporters and individual supporters do not have voting rights.

MedVirginia

Michael Matthews, CEO, MedVirginia

MedVirgina is a Limited Liability Company (LLC). There is a five-member board of managers consisting of four physicians and a CIO of a major health system. The governing board members have been the same since the organization was formed. Michael Matthews, CEO, believes that the key to their success is that they pay attention to "bottom line results," and they are able to meet strategic priorities. He believes that having a small board means that they can be very responsive to issues as they arise.

In addition to the five-member board, there is a Board Advisory Council whose members include representation from:
- Virginia Department of Health
- Virginia Hospital and Healthcare Association
- Hospitals
- Free clinics
- Community agencies
- Lewis Sullivan, Secretary of HHS under President George H. W. Bush

The board convenes ad hoc groups for specific projects to ensure that all key stakeholders are involved and to ensure that recommendations are well vetted.

Rochester RHIO—Rochester, New York

Ted Kremer, Executive Director, Rochester RHIO

According to Ted Kremer, Executive Director, the board of the Rochester RHIO consists of member representation including:
- Three hospital systems
- One hospital
- Three health plans
- Department of Health
- Medical Society of Monroe County
- Consumer Advocate
- Legal Action Group
- Chamber of Commerce

The board chair is head of the Rochester Chamber of Commerce, and the members of the board are all decision makers in their own organizations with titles such as chief medical information officer, chief medical officer, executive vice president, etc. Kremer believes that it is vital to have people on the board who can speak for their organizations.

Nebraska Health Information Initiative (NeHII)

Deb Bass, Executive Director, Nebraska Health Information Initiative

Nebraska has taken a somewhat different approach to their board from many of the other organizations we interviewed. Deb Bass, Executive Director of NeHII, describes how the board seats are related to the type of membership an organization holds.

There are two classes of membership in NeHII. Class A Collaborative members are generally individuals and are representatives from physician or consumer groups. They pay $100 per year to have the privilege to elect two Class A members to the board. Class B membership is comprised of healthcare organizations that make a larger financial commitment. This can range from $25,000 to upwards of $250,000.

The board members are allocated one vote for each dollar contributed to elect future board members.

There are four standing members appointed to the board:
- Consumer advocate
- State government representative currently filled by the lt. governor who is the state's HIT Coordinator
- NeHII Executive Director
- Representative from the Nebraska Hospital Association

Additional board seats may be filled by 16 Class B members and 2 Class A members.

Indiana Health Information Technology Corporation (IHIT Corp.)

David Johnson, President and CEO, BioCrossroads

In Indiana, the organization responsible for statewide HIE efforts is the Indiana Health Information Technology Corporation (IHIT Corp). This is a not-for-profit corporation.

The board of IHIT Corp. consists of representatives from multiple public and private organizations which include:
- Indiana Secretary of Family and Social Services Agency
- Indiana Commissioner of Public Health
- Indiana Secretary of Commerce
- Director of Indiana OMB (Office of Management and Budget)
- Interagency State Council on Minority Health
- Indiana Hospitals
- Licensed physician
- One disproportionate share hospital
- Rural health representative
- Consumers
- Research scientist
- Expert on data privacy and security

In addition to the board, there are several Advisory Councils:
- HIE policy and technical advisory
- Data provision and use

- Patient advocacy
- Research and education

CareSpark

Liesa Jenkins, Executive Director, CareSpark

According to Liesa Jenkins, Executive Director of CareSpark, their board comprises between nine and fifteen individuals who are committed to the mission of the organization and are willing to put that commitment above their own personal or organizational agenda.

The philosophy of the board is to create an environment in which the expectation is that "The board is in place to work for the good of all. Individual organizations may get some incidental benefit from the work as well, but the only way for anyone to benefit is if everybody wins."

CareSpark has been very deliberate about the composition of the board and uses a matrix approach to determine who is nominated to serve on the board. They believe that it is crucial to have a good mix of perspectives and skills represented. To ensure a good balance on the board, when considering potential board members, they consider the following principles:

- Stakeholder perspectives:
  They ensure that there are people who can communicate well with hospitals, physicians, payers, consumers, and other stakeholders.
- Geographic and demographic representation:
  They ensure that the representation reflects the regions they serve, as two-thirds of their patients reside in Tennessee and one-third resides in Virginia.
- Skill sets:
  The skill sets and experience that they look for among the group of board members include:
  - Good public speaker
  - Good with legal and contractual issues
  - Experience in budget, finance, and fundraising
  - Technical understanding
  - Clinicians
  - Facilitator/meeting leader
  - Public relations experience
  - Internal operations knowledge
  - Personnel management experience

There are four to five ongoing committees that are open to anyone who expresses an interest in participating and contributing. Committee members are expected to be active, contribute a great deal of effort, and have expertise in the relevant areas. These committees make recommendations to the board.

New Mexico Health Information Collaborative (NMHIC)

Jeff Blair, Director of Health Informatics, LCF Research, New Mexico Health Information Collaborative

According to Jeff Blair, Director of Health Informatics at LCF Research (the not-for-profit that created, staffs, and operates NMHIC), a new expanded Board of Directors was formed in early 2010 to preside over LCF Research, including the research and NMHIC divisions.[5] This board includes:

- State HIT Coordinator/CIO of NM Department of Health
- Deputy Director of Medicaid
- Four directors representing medical practices
- Five directors from a large medical group
- Five directors from hospitals
- Seven directors from health plans
- One from the Quality Improvement Organization
- Four from the University of New Mexico
- Two from laboratories
- Two from major community employers
- One from wellness and preventive education
- One from applied health research
- One representing consumers
- One representing rural telehealth

This board is in the process of selecting the committee members who will provide governance that more directly impacts the organization.

Michigan Health Information Network (MiHIN)

Beth Nagel, Health Information Technology Coordinator, Michigan Department of Community Health

The following guiding principles are based on the experience Michigan gained through the MiHIN *Conduit to Care* process and have been updated to reflect the current state-wide and national HIT and HIE landscape. These guiding principles will serve as the foundation for the Governance of the MiHIN.

Guiding Principle 1: Michigan citizens are at the center of the MiHIN goals to improve patient care and population health.

Health information exchange in Michigan will be designed to benefit Michigan residents. Consumer privacy, security, and confidentiality are paramount and as such, the MiHIN will adhere to all federal and state laws regarding privacy and security to build trust.

Guiding Principle 2: The MiHIN will leverage existing and planned information technology.

Health information exchange will be made accessible to all naturally occurring and commerce-defined communities of providers by leveraging—and to the extent possible not duplicating—existing and planned information technology investments by the state of Michigan, regional, community, private and other HIE initiatives.

Guiding Principle 3: Multi-stakeholder collaboration is needed to implement achievable and measurable initiatives.

Cooperation and collaboration on the implementation of health information exchange will drive innovation and change across the various stakeholders in the state, as well as foster the sustainability and financial solvency of statewide HIE efforts.

Guiding Principle 4: The MiHIN will conform to applicable federal guidelines.

Statewide health information exchange will be designed and implemented to support Michigan priorities within the guidelines of the Office of the National Coordinator— Meaningful Use, standards, NHIN, etc.—in order to facilitate national health exchange and optimize funding.

Guiding Principle 5: Those that benefit should participate in paying the cost.

Long-term financial sustainability of the MiHIN will be dependent upon fair contribution from those who benefit.

Guiding Principle 6: Adoption and use of the MiHIN is critical to success.

Since the benefit of statewide health information exchange comes from adoption and use, the MiHIN should be attractive to a broad range of healthcare stakeholders throughout Michigan and be designed and implemented in phases to deliver early results to support increased adoption.

RESOURCES

Colorado Regional Health Information Organization (CORHIO) Committees. http://www.corhio.org/ About/Committees.htm. Accessed April, 2010.

Jenkins L. CareSpark: Redwood Health Information Collaborative. Presented February 18, 2009. http:// www.mendocinohre.org/rhic/200902/CareSpark_2-18-09.ppt. Accessed April, 2010.

HealthBridge. HealthBridge Profile. http://www.healthbridge.org/index.php?option=com_content&task= view&id=5&Itemid=6. Accessed April, 2010.

Vermont Information Technology Leaders (VITL). About Us. http://www.vitl.net/interior.php/pid/2. Accessed April, 2010.

MedVirginia. About MedVirginia. http://www.medvirginia.net/about.html. Accessed April, 2010.

NC HIE Sustainability Plan: http://www.nchica.org/HIT_HIE/NHIN2/Sustainability%20Plan.pdf.

Toolkit for State-Level HIE: http://www.nchica.org/About/toolkit.htm.

ARRA HITECH Resources: http://www.nchica.org/HIT_HIE/ARRA.htm.

Louisville Health Information Exchange. Bylaws of Louisville Health Information Exchange, Inc. http:// www.louhie.org/Downloads/LouHIE%20ByLaws%203-24-06.DOC. Accessed April, 2010.

Bronx RHIO. By-Laws of Bronx RHIO, Inc. https://www.bronxrhio.net/images/downloads/BronxRHIO_ By-Laws_9-24-2007.pdf. Accessed April ,2010.

U.S. Treasury, Department of the IRS. Exemption Requirements - Section 501(c)3 Organizations. http:// www.irs.gov/charities/charitable/article/0,,id=96099,00.html. Accessed April, 2010.

U.S. Treasury, Department of the IRS. Regional Health Information Organization (RHIO) Frequently Asked Questions. http://www.irs.gov/charities/charitable/article/0,,id=206129,00.html. Accessed April, 2010.

U.S. Treasury, Department of the IRS. State Links (A collection of links to state government web sites with useful information for tax-exempt organizations.) http://www.irs.gov/charities/article/0,,id=129028,00. html. Accessed April, 2010.

Department of Health & Human Services. Sample Business Associate Contract Provisions. Posted August 14, 2002. http://www.hhs.gov/ocr/privacy/hipaa/understanding/coveredentities/contractprov. html. Accessed November, 2009.

NHIN Cooperative DURSA Workgroup. (2009, January 23). Draft Data Use and Reciprocal Support Agreement (DURSA). http://healthit.hhs.gov/portal/server.pt/gateway/PTARGS_0_10731_849891_0_0_ 18/DRAFT%20NHIN%20Trial%20Implementations%20Production%20DURSA-3.pdf. Accessed November, 2009.

Arizona Health-e Connection. Model Health Information Exchange Participation Agreement. http://www. azgita.gov/ehealth/hispc/AzHECmodelHIEparticipation.pdf. Accessed November, 2009.

Markle Foundation. Connecting for Health: M2 A Model Contract for Health Information Exchange. http://www.connectingforhealth.org/commonframework/#guide. Accessed November, 2009.

Bronx Regional Health Information Organization (Bronx RHIO). Policies and Procedures. http://www. bronxrhio.org/downloads/BronxRHIO_PoliciesAndProcedures_April08.pdf. Accessed November, 2009.

California Regional Health Information Organization (CalRHIO). Business Associate Agreement Template. http://www.calrhio.org/crweb-files/docs-hietools/Business_Associate_Agreement_Template.doc. Accessed April, 2010.

Other sample agreements can also be accessed from the CalRHIO website:

Data Sharing Agreement: http://www.calrhio.org/crweb-files/docs-hietools/Information_Sharing_ Agreement.pdf. Accessed September, 2010.

Participation Agreement:http://www.calrhio.org/crweb-files/docs-hietools/Participation_Agreement_ DWT.pdf. Accessed September, 2010.

Memorandum of Understanding Template: http://www.calrhio.org/crweb-files/docs-hietools/MOU_ Template.doc. Accessed September, 2010.

REFERENCES

1. Department of Health & Human Services, Office of the National Coordinator for Health Information Technology. State Health Information Exchange Cooperative Agreement Program, Funding Opportunity Announcement, 2009; 15. http://healthit.hhs.gov/portal/server.pt/gateway/PTARGS_0_10741_ 888442_0_0_18/FOA_State%20Health%20Information%20Exchange%20Cooperative%20Agreement %20Program_Sept3_updated%20funding%20formula.doc. Accessed April, 2010.

2. Department of Health & Human Services, Office of the National Coordinator for Health Information Technology. 2010 Consumer Consent Options for Electronic HIE: Policy Considerations and Analysis, retrieved from. http://healthit.hhs.gov/portal/server.pt/gateway/PTARGS_0.../ ChoiceModelFinal_11673_911197_0_0_18/ChoiceModelFinal032610.pdf. Accessed April, 2010.

3. Privacy and security Tiger Team http://healthit.hhs.gov/portal/server.pt?open=512&mode=2&objID =2833&PageID=19421Accessed September, 2010.

4. NHIN Cooperative DURSA Team. 2009 Data Use and Reciprocal Support Agreement (DURSA) For NHIN Limited Production Pilot Activities, retrieved from http://healthit.hhs.gov/portal/server.pt/ gateway/PTARGS_0_11673_909240_0_0_18/DURSAVersionforProductionPilotsFinal.pdf. Accessed April, 2010.

5. New Mexico State HIE Strategic and Operational Plan. www.nmhic.org. Accessed September, 2010.

CHAPTER 5

Creating Your Strategic Plan

"Make no little plans; They have no magic
to stir men's blood."

Daniel H. Burnham
Architect of the Chicago World's Fair

INTRODUCTION

This chapter is about how to develop your Strategic Plan. This is not a primer on how to write the perfect plan; there are already many available resources for that. Here, we discuss an approach to identifying and addressing the key issues and decisions that you will grapple with on your journey to building an HIE.

The Strategic Plan is the foundation for the formation and development of your organization, and it serves many purposes. Start your Strategic Plan early in your development. You will refer to it often.

The collaborative process is essential in developing your Strategic Plan, and broad, active stakeholder input is critical. An open process provides the opportunity for the leaders of the community and the HIE Board to work together to build consensus, and it stimulates both understanding and buy-in for how your HIE will reach its objectives. This collaborative process establishes a solid foundation for securing continued stakeholder engagement and participation. "Never take your stakeholders for granted," advises Laura Adams, President & CEO, Rhode Island Quality Institute.

Once written, a well-documented Strategic Plan will help keep the organization focused and provide a point of reference for decision making. It contains your Vision and Mission Statements and describes the approach you are going to use to accomplish your mission. The Strategic Plan also includes your organization's objectives, and it creates the roadmap to your desired future by describing the specific initiatives that you plan to undertake to accomplish those objectives. For that reason, a Strategic Plan is also referred to by many consultants as a "strategy and roadmap."

COMPONENTS OF THE STRATEGIC PLAN

There are wide varieties of approaches to developing a Strategic Plan, and there are almost as many terms for the various components as there are consultants in the field.

Components of a Strategic Plan

1. Organization and Environment Assessment

2. Vision

3. Mission

4. Principles/Core Values

5. Objectives

6. Strategies

7. Initiatives

8. Evaluation and Measurement Criteria

Figure 5-1: Components of a Strategic Plan

Figure 5-1 identifies the key components we use in our firm to describe a good Strategic Plan. In this chapter we provide guidance as you work through the various strategic plan components that are necessary for you to clarify what your HIE organization needs to become.

Thanks to the U.S. Department of Health & Human Services' State HIE Cooperative Agreement Program, funded through the HITECH Act, there are many good examples of HIE strategic plans publically available. Every state was required to submit a state HIE strategic plan as a requirement to receive funding. Consider reviewing some of these plans. You should definitely review and be familiar with your own state's plan. See the Resources section at the end of this chapter for links to some of the state HIE strategic plans.

We start this discussion by defining the various components of the Strategic Plan. Further in this chapter, we discuss each in more detail.

Organization and Environment Assessment

In Chapter 2, *Getting Started*, we discussed your initial scan of the community. You will use that information, and more, as you develop your objectives, create your strategies to achieve your objectives, and define the specific initiatives that you will need to undertake to achieve your objectives. At a minimum, you need to know the types and numbers of healthcare providers in your community, have a sense of the rate of EHR adoption, and the overall knowledge level of—and perspectives on—HIE. You will also include your organization's structure and other relevant information.

Vision and Mission Statements

In Chapter 3, *Navigating Your Early Stage Formation*, we discussed two essential elements that are required in your Strategic Plan—developing your Vision and Mission Statements. If you have not already developed your Vision and Mission Statements, please return to Chapter 3, *Navigating Your Early Stage Formation* and complete that work before you begin working on the rest of your plan.

As a reminder, we restate the definitions of vision and mission here.

Vision Statement: Your Vision Statement should describe your view of a desired future state. Make this future-oriented and inspirational from the perspective of your organization. It describes the future you see.

Mission Statement: Your Mission Statement describes the fundamental purpose for which your organization exists. While the Mission Statement should stretch you, it also needs to fall within the realm of being achievable.

Two comments about your Mission Statement. First, it will probably change over time as the needs of your community change. Second, it should always be congruent with your vision. The relationship between the two is straightforward. By accomplishing your mission, you will be contributing to the fulfillment of your vision. Review your Vision and Mission Statements and refer to them frequently as you work through developing the rest of the Strategic Plan.

Objectives

Objectives are statements that either describe the presence of a significant artifact(s), such as a document containing a list of approved privacy policies, or the evidence of a significant capability, such as the ability to connect to the NHIN. Typically, a completed objective is considered a milestone. Objectives are *what* you want to accomplish.

Strategies

Strategies are documented in the form of statements that describe the approach that you will use to accomplish one or more of your objectives. Strategic statements describe, at a high level, *how* you will go about achieving your objectives.

Initiatives

An initiative can be thought of as a project or a grouping of related activities and resources that, when completed, accomplish one or more of your objectives. Typically, when forming an HIE, there are a number of initiatives underway concurrently. Generally, but not always, initiatives will be domain-specific.

Evaluation and Measurement Criteria

Measurements relate to the steps involved in accomplishing your objectives and provide a means to determine when those objectives have been met. They define what needs to be accomplished and by when. They enable you to track and report on your progress.

As we stated earlier, developing your Strategic Plan is an iterative process and involves revisiting the key components often. Why? As your organization grows and matures, you will typically add new objectives. Strategic planning, like stakeholder engagement, is an ongoing activity. Figure 5-2 depicts how these components keep driving each other to ensure that all sections of your Strategic Plan are in alignment.

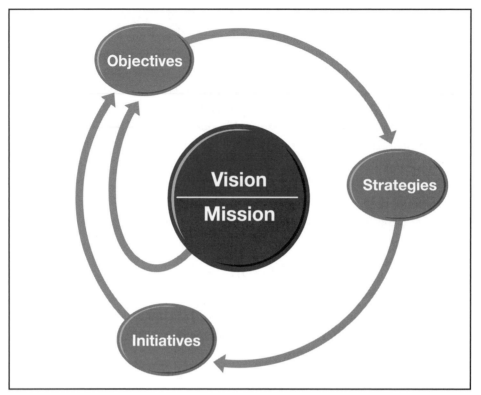

Figure 5-2: Drivers of a Strategic Plan. © 2009 Mosaica Partners, LLC. Used by permission.

DEVELOPING YOUR STRATEGIC PLAN

The following section discusses developing each of the components of your strategic plan and includes:

1. Creating your Vision Statement
2. Creating your Mission Statement
3. Identifying your principles/core values
4. Developing your initial objectives
5. Creating your strategic approach
6. Defining your initiatives
7. Establishing your evaluation and measurement criteria

Creating Your Vision and Mission Statements

We discussed creating your Vision and Mission Statements in Chapter 3, *Navigating Your Early Stage Formation*. Please refer back to that chapter for our suggested approach.

Identifying Your Principles/Core Values

Your values and principles state clearly and concisely the basis upon which your organization is founded and will operate. These principles form the foundation for all of your decisions and they will permeate your policies and activities.

Your core values communicate to the outside world who you are and how you conduct business. They help stakeholders understand your organization, determine if they want to interact with you, and how much they can trust you.

To identify your principles, begin by brainstorming your beliefs and what you feel is important. Identify key words and phrases that describe how, as an organization, you will interact with the community and conduct your business.

Developing Your Initial Objectives

As mentioned earlier, objectives are statements that describe the presence of either artifacts (significant items) or capabilities that you will need to achieve your mission. Objectives should be clearly worded so that you can assess whether or not they have been achieved. Your workgroups will each contribute to defining and achieving your initial objectives. Examples of objectives include:

- We have a business plan that has been approved by the board.
- We have developed a clear statement of how we will ensure the privacy and security of patient information before we begin operations.
- We have the ability to connect to NHIN.
- We have the ability to continually monitor the community's wants and needs and to translate them into a list of specific services that they desire.
- We have the ability to continually assess community wants and needs, the HIE's financial condition, and any new statutes and regulations to determine—in a structured manner—which activities the HIE should undertake and in which order.

Creating Your Strategies

Strategies identify the specific approaches that you will use to reach your objectives. The strategic approaches are often what change the most as the organization matures in its strategic planning, learns more about its environment, and adds capabilities. To create your strategies, the question you need to answer is, "In what manner will we go about achieving our objective(s)?"

We recommend that your strategy be stated in the form of declarative sentences. There may be a single statement or a list of strategy statements. Collectively, these statements describe the strategic approach that you plan to use to accomplish your objectives and thus achieve your mission.

Strategy is developed and refined as you define your specific objectives. The planning and review process is cyclic. Once you agree on an objective, give some thought to the high-level approach most appropriate to achieve that objective. Those approaches are woven into the overall strategic approach you will adopt. Example strategy statements are provided below.

- We place a high priority on going live quickly with a minimum set of services, as opposed to taking longer and going live with a more complete set of services.
- We will utilize external consultants and subject matter experts (SMEs) to assist us in reaching our objectives.

- We will, to the extent possible, utilize the services of our State Designated Entity to provide us with the essential policies and agreements required to operate an HIE in this state.
- We will utilize volunteer help from our own community to perform all tasks, as opposed to using outside assistance.
- We will utilize the technical infrastructure of [Vendor X] on a shared basis to provide services to our community.
- We will build our own HIE technical infrastructure using open source components.

The totality of the agreed upon strategies is referred to as your strategic approach.

Defining Your Initiatives

Initiatives are the specific projects that, when completed in harmony with your strategic approach, will enable your organization's objectives to be met.

Designing your initiatives is both an art and a science.

First, determine what objectives need to be accomplished. Second, identify the activities you need to perform to move you closer to achieving your objectives. The activities you identify can then be grouped into logical clusters. These logical groupings of activities become your initiatives.

An initiative may address a specific objective or it may address more than one objective. For example, the initiative, "Locate, secure, and prepare a physical facility from which the HIE will operate" will involve activities in both the Business & Finance and the Technology & Security domains: Business & Finance because it involves business planning and signing contracts and Technology & Security because it involves the physical area that will be used to house any required technology and must be in conformance with previously agreed upon security requirements and technology best practices.

Ensure that specific action plans exist and are incorporated into each initiative. Initiatives can be further divided into phases such as short-term initiatives (6–9 months for completion) or longer term (10–14 months). Developing your initiatives is an interactive process that should include your key stakeholders and your workgroups.

Examples of initiatives are as follows:

- Prepare a business plan for approval by the board.
- Locate and hire an executive director.
- Understand and document the security and confidentiality requirements that must be accommodated by our technical infrastructure before we can go live.
- Locate, secure, and prepare a physical facility from which the HIE will operate.

Establishing Your Evaluation and Measurement Criteria

You need to be able to gauge your progress toward reaching each of your defined objectives. To do this in a structured way, you should identify intermediate steps and success criteria to help you determine the status of an objective or when an objective has been accomplished. Also include a date by which those criteria should be met.

Examples of measures are shown below:

- Assign a sub team to locate and recommend a physical site by June 30.
- Site selection team to have developed consolidated requirements list by July 15.
- Site selection team to have viewed possible conforming sites by August 12.
- Site selection team to make recommendation of primary and two alternative sites to board by August 30.
- Board to decide on most appropriate site and begin negotiations by September 16.
- Take possession of site by October 3.

What about Goals?

We have consistently used the term *objectives* in this chapter. But what about goals? Some people may consider the terms interchangeable. We do not. We view goal statements as describing a specific thing to be done by a specific time. As such, they could relate to either objectives or initiatives.

As we have previously stated, there are many opinions as to how to define the various terms. To reduce confusion, we explain next how we define and use the terms *objectives* and *goals* in our practice as HIE consultants and in this book.

Viewed from the perspective of an objective, a goal could describe a point along the way to developing an artifact or a capability. For example, in the objective, "We have a business plan that has been approved by the board," a goal could be to have a first draft by October 23. That could have been preceded by the goal, "Identify someone to lead the business plan writing effort by August 15."

Viewed from the perspective of an initiative, a goal could describe the completion of a specific phase, activity, or task associated with that initiative. For example, in the initiative, "Locate and hire an Executive Director," a goal could be to have decided on a short list of final candidates by March 22. Another goal could be, "Make an offer to the leading candidate by April 3."

Whom to Involve in This Activity

Your board members and your workgroups will be key contributors to creating your strategic plan. As mentioned earlier, in Chapter 4, *Establish a Formal Organizational Governance Structure*, the workgroups should comprise individuals with the skills and expertise relevant to the workgroup to which they are assigned. It is also important to ensure that there is broad community representation in, and support for, your strategic planning efforts.

You may want to consider hiring a professional facilitator to assist you in developing your strategic plan. In addition to facilitation skills, you will need to involve SMEs in the area of HIE formation. These are people with in-depth knowledge of HIEs and the capabilities, processes, and resources required to develop a successful HIE.

If your state's State Designated Entity is operational, consider including a representative from that group as well as a representative from your area's Regional Extension Center. If you are the organization charged with planning your state HIE, it is critical to involve stakeholders from multiple regions of the state in your planning. You need to ensure that your plan considers your state's demographic and community diversity. You

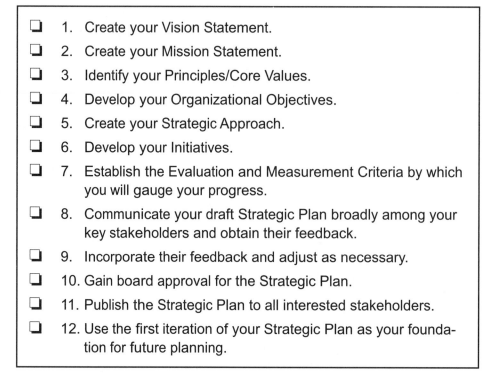

❏   1. Create your Vision Statement.

❏   2. Create your Mission Statement.

❏   3. Identify your Principles/Core Values.

❏   4. Develop your Organizational Objectives.

❏   5. Create your Strategic Approach.

❏   6. Develop your Initiatives.

❏   7. Establish the Evaluation and Measurement Criteria by which you will gauge your progress.

❏   8. Communicate your draft Strategic Plan broadly among your key stakeholders and obtain their feedback.

❏   9. Incorporate their feedback and adjust as necessary.

❏   10. Gain board approval for the Strategic Plan.

❏   11. Publish the Strategic Plan to all interested stakeholders.

❏   12. Use the first iteration of your Strategic Plan as your foundation for future planning.

Figure 5-3: Checklist—Developing Your Strategic Plan

also need to ensure that your state's plan is aligned with the nationwide HIE framework, plan, and objectives, as well as with other states' plans.

Figure 5-3 contains a checklist that identifies many of the activities and steps needed to develop your Strategic Plan.

CHAPTER SUMMARY

When properly completed, the Vision and Mission Statements, the objectives, the strategic approach(es), the initiatives, and the evaluation and measurement criteria form a congruent whole. This is your Strategic Plan.

In this chapter, we have covered creating your Strategic Plan. The components include your Vision and Mission Statements, which are used to develop the objectives for what you need to accomplish for your HIE to fulfill its mission. Your strategies describe the approaches you will use to reach your objectives.

After you conduct a gap analysis between where you are today and where you need to be, you will develop specific initiatives to close these gaps. Initiatives are the projects that enable your objectives to be met. Finally, you create measurements that will help you gauge your progress towards meeting your objectives.

When you complete the activities in this chapter, you will have developed your Strategic Plan.

RESOURCES
State HIE Plans

California Strategic Plan: California Health & Human Services Agency. CA Health Information Exchange (HIE) Plan. http://www.hie.ca.gov/HIEPlan/tabid/72/Default.aspx. Accessed November, 2009.

Maryland HIE Strategic and Operational Plan. http://mhcc.maryland.gov/electronichealth/hiestateplan/hit_state_plan_060910.pdf. Accessed September, 2010.

New Hampshire Strategic Plan: New Hampshire Citizens Health Initiative. A Strategic Plan for Health Information Technology and Exchange. http://steppingupnh.org.

New Mexico HIE Strategic and Operational Plan. http://www.nmhic.org. Accessed September, 2010.

New York eHealth Collaborative State HIE Strategic Plan. http://www.health.state.ny.us/funding/rfa/0903160302/health_it_strategic_plan.pdf.

Tennessee Draft HIE Strategic Plan. http://www.tennesseeanytime.org/ehealth/documents/TennesseeHIEStrategicPlanFinal10-12-09_000.pdf. Accessed September, 2010.

Utah Strategic Plan. http://health.utah.gov/phi/ehealth/UT_HIE_StrategicPlans_March2010.pdf. Accessed September, 2010.

Other Resources

Thornewill J, Baluch J, Cox B, Dowling A, Sudol R. Stakeholder Research Report 2007. Posted December 14, 2007. http://www.louhie.org/Downloads/LouHIE%20research%20report%20v8%20final.pdf. Accessed November, 2009.

AHRQ. Health IT Survey Compendium. http://healthit.ahrq.gov/portal/server.pt?open=512&objID=653&&PageID=12713&mode=2&in_hi_userid=3882&cached=true. Accessed November, 2009.

http://www.unh.edu/chi/media/Reports/2009StrategicPlan_Web.pdf. Accessed November, 2009.

McNamara C. Strategic Planning (in Nonprofit or For-Profit Organizations). 1997.

http://managementhelp.org/plan_dec/str_plan/str_plan.htm. Accessed November, 2009.

CHAPTER 6

Your Business Plan Defines How Delivering Value Drives Your Sustainability

"You need to run the Health Information Exchange like a business; But do it in the best interest of patient care."

John Kansky
Vice President—Business Development
Indiana Health Information Exchange

INTRODUCTION

A Business Plan is the management tool that describes what you will do to achieve your mission and how your organization will meet its objectives. It also serves as a useful document for the management team and the board in communicating the HIE's plans and direction—thus effectively ensuring that all participants are collectively focused on the organization's agreed upon mission and the agreed upon approach to reach that mission.

The inherent value of a Business Plan is that it encourages you to think carefully about the business of health information exchange and how you will translate your mission into an operational reality. In this chapter, we discuss the key issues and decisions you will grapple with as you move forward in building an HIE in which your stakeholders will want to participate and one they will help you sustain. We focus on ensuring that every part of your Business Plan moves you toward sustainability—a critical component that has proven to be elusive to many early HIE efforts. As Dick Thompson, Executive Director/CEO, Quality Health Network, points out, you need to "understand that there are many points of value. Don't hang all your efforts on one hook [service]. And realize that there is more than one way that people can perceive value."

ENGAGING STAKEHOLDERS

It is imperative that your business model be based upon—and be congruent with—the concept of *mutually agreed upon exchanges of value*. An essential question your business/financial model must answer is, "What services do our stakeholders want and

> What services do our stakeholders want and need us to provide and how much are they willing to pay for those services?

need us to provide; and how much will they be willing to pay for providing those services?" We believe that answering this question is the basis of a solid, sustainable HIE business plan. "[You] need to build the social capital. Financial capital follows the social capital," says Laura Adams, President & CEO, Rhode Island Quality Institute. "[There is] no substitute for going through the process yourself. Don't assume you can avoid the community engagement process. Financial capital won't buy you social capital, but it can fool you into thinking you don't need it."

You will be able to construct a solid Business Plan—that is both appropriate and financially sustainable—only after you have (1) defined your HIE in terms of the services that provide value to your stakeholders; and (2) developed a viable approach to delivering those services.

Stakeholders need to believe that the HIE can provide them with real value. Until they do, they generally don't show much interest in the details of how the services will be delivered or about the various aspects of HIE business models. It can be difficult to get them engaged. However, that will change as you actively seek their input, and they realize that you are truly interested in meeting *their* needs.

The effort involved in getting your stakeholders to the point where they realize that the HIE can provide them with valuable capabilities or services is an essential component of the stakeholder engagement process. When your stakeholders are truly engaged, not only will they be intrigued about your HIE and the improved capabilities and outcomes it can provide them, they often will care enough to become more actively involved—including actively participating in a dialog with you or even asking how they can support your efforts.

This participation can only be achieved through an understanding of, and delivering on, stakeholder-defined value. As mentioned earlier, forming an HIE is, in consulting parlance, a large change management project. Understanding stakeholder values and acting upon that understanding is consistent with the discipline of change management, which is based on the premise that when people or organizations value something, there is the potential that they will change their behavior to receive it, including paying for it. Conversely, if they do not see appropriate value, they will resist any change to the status quo.

Just as in developing your strategic plan, developing a business plan is an interactive and iterative process with your stakeholders. You need input and recommendations from each of the workgroups participating in your HIE formation efforts. If done correctly, they will form their recommendations based upon input, feedback, and involvement from your stakeholders.

Understanding the impact of HIE on your stakeholders—from the perspective of both value and cost—will provide you with a framework for developing business value propositions for each of your various stakeholder segments. It will also help you identify areas in which there may be barriers to HIE adoption that need your specific attention. Such an understanding can also point to factors that are critical to your success.

An innovative approach to stakeholder involvement can be seen in Central Illinois. According to Joy Duling, Project Director for HIE and the Regional Extension Center at Quality Quest for Health of Illinois, her organization began by gathering all those who worked on HIE councils and workgroups, plus anyone else interested in the HIE movement, into the Central Illinois HIE Alliance. This group will evolve into an organization and participation structure as the HIE effort matures.

Why Understanding Value Is Important to HIE Sustainability

An observation related by Laura Kolkman that illustrates careful thinking is of attending a session to report on the results of the first set of NHIN initiatives back in 2005. The presenters were great people with good credentials and abundant experience. Having just formed her own consulting firm, she sat in the audience a bit in awe of the presenters who represented the well-known organizations that had participated in these projects. After all, the federal government had chosen them to deliver on an important set of objectives. As you may recall, one of the objectives each project team was required to address was an approach to financial sustainability. As she sat there listening to the various presentations, the thought struck her that none of the teams had been able to demonstrate a reasonable sustainability model for a nationwide HIE.

She began to think about why all these talented people, working together, had not come up with a model that would provide financial sustainability for the NHIN or HIE. "What," she wondered, "is preventing the creation of a solid approach to HIE sustainability?" She thought about how businesses in general become financially sustainable—what was required? Certainly, to be financially sustainable, a business needs a good return on its investment. To get that return, it needs ongoing sources of funds—a revenue stream. In that context, she then thought, "OK, so what's necessary in the marketplace to generate revenue?" *Answer*: "Demand for the product or service that meets a need."

There are many unmet needs in our world. Some could provide good sources of revenue and some would not. What's the difference? Why do most HIEs have such a problem with this formula and with positive outcome? Health information exchange certainly addresses an unmet need. We cannot effectively share health information today (2005), and it is generally recognized that healthcare would benefit from electronically collecting and sharing patient information. Hmmm.

Then it came to her. The missing piece was that no one was able to identify the *value* that their models would deliver. They had not been able to quantify the value that the HIE services would provide to their stakeholders. There was little demand for HIE because HIEs were not delivering services that provided a recognized value to their stakeholders. The stakeholders weren't interested, and they certainly weren't excited.

What she finally realized is illustrated in Figure 6-1.

RECOGNIZED VALUE!

An HIE needs to provide value that is recognized and appreciated by its stakeholders. Only their opinion

> What was missing in the NHIN scenario was providing *recognized value* to a base of stakeholders.

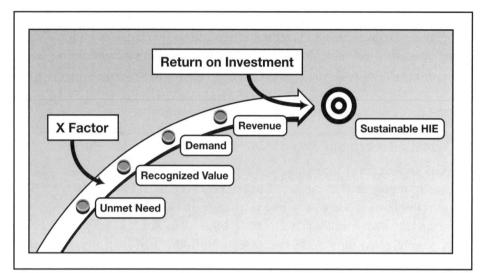

Figure 6-1: Finding the Value. © 2007 Mosaica Partners, LLC. Used by permission.

counts. The services the HIE offers must address its stakeholders' problems (pain points) and provide them value—value for which they are willing to change their behavior and even pay.

In business, it's all about providing value to your customers, clients, or patients. In the HIE business, it is all about providing value to your stakeholders and, in doing so, improving the quality of healthcare.

Three Reasons Why Understanding Stakeholder Value Is Important to an HIE

1. You will understand what they will change their behavior for.

2. You will understand what services your stakeholders may be willing to pay for.

3. It will help you determine and prioritize which services and the order in which your HIE should provide them.

When you understand what your stakeholders value, you gain insight into at least three important areas that are required for sustainability.

First, by understanding what your stakeholders value, you will understand what may cause them to change their behavior. What value will it take to motivate them to modify their existing work processes to include the sharing of patient information? The key to your success is designing your business and services around what your stakeholders value. As often mentioned in this book, building an HIE is a change management project, and change is typically difficult for us humans. We like the status quo. Our bodies continually seek homeostasis—that *even* balance. Any change puts us off balance. However, it is well-known that, generally, we willingly change for something that we value and deem worth the effort or cost.

Second, you will begin to understand, at a high level, what services those stakeholders may be willing to pay for—if they find *enough* value.

And *third*, identifying what your stakeholders value, and how they prioritize that value, helps you determine the order in which your HIE should introduce services. You cannot introduce every service on day one. You need to prioritize them. This prioritization process informs your business plan.

Of the many segments of stakeholders, we believe that physicians and hospitals are two of the most important and influential stakeholder segments, especially during the formation stage of an HIE. You must engage representatives of these groups early—and often. For obvious reasons, their buy-in and participation is critical for the success of your HIE. Be proactive. Never take your stakeholders' support for granted.

Leaders of successful HIE efforts realize that you've got to have a WIN early—one that your stakeholders perceive as a win—no matter how small. They say that it's best to start small and be successful—and then add layers of complexity, rather than try for too much, too soon. Failures happen with big, complex endeavors.

Understanding Stakeholder Defined Value

The first step to financial stability, then, is to understand how your stakeholders define value as it relates to HIE. Each community is unique in its culture and the nuances of its values. An in-depth understanding of your community is necessary, not only to determine the services that you will offer, but it also informs the type of governance that is right for the community, the fee structures that are appropriate for the stakeholders, and how the overall mission and guiding principles of the HIE will be implemented. All of these should directly relate to what your stakeholders have told you they value.

The best approach to understand what your stakeholders value, in relation to health information exchange, is to simply ask them directly. Ask them, from their perspective, what is important and what is a priority for them.

Many times organizations fail in this first critical step of directly engaging physicians and hospitals and, instead, believe that others can speak for these groups. While surrogates, such as professional association representatives, may be able to accurately convey the opinions of these stakeholder segments, they cannot replace direct stakeholder engagement.

> It is imperative that your business model be based on—and be congruent with—the concept of *mutually agreed upon exchanges of value*.

There are two key reasons why you need to speak directly to your stakeholders. First, of course, you want their perspectives. However, even more importantly, you want to demonstrate your commitment to doing the right thing the right way. When you talk to them directly, they understand that you are willing to listen to them and hear what *they* have to say. They feel they are a part of the process. They are actively *participating*. There is no shortcut or substitute for direct stakeholder participation and dialogue.

The Dialogue with Stakeholders to Understand What They Value

Engaging in an ongoing, long-running dialogue with your stakeholders is critical. It is a two-way communication. You receive their perspectives and, in turn, you provide information on the project—and how you are using their input. Use the information they provide and then communicate back to them with messages that show you are listening to them and interested in what they have to say.

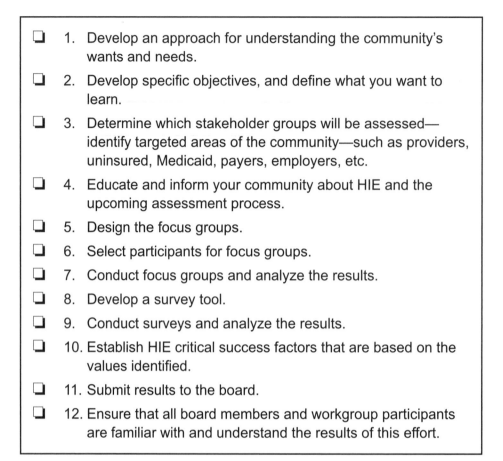

❏   1. Develop an approach for understanding the community's wants and needs.

❏   2. Develop specific objectives, and define what you want to learn.

❏   3. Determine which stakeholder groups will be assessed—identify targeted areas of the community—such as providers, uninsured, Medicaid, payers, employers, etc.

❏   4. Educate and inform your community about HIE and the upcoming assessment process.

❏   5. Design the focus groups.

❏   6. Select participants for focus groups.

❏   7. Conduct focus groups and analyze the results.

❏   8. Develop a survey tool.

❏   9. Conduct surveys and analyze the results.

❏ 10. Establish HIE critical success factors that are based on the values identified.

❏ 11. Submit results to the board.

❏ 12. Ensure that all board members and workgroup participants are familiar with and understand the results of this effort.

Figure 6-2: Checklist—Understanding Stakeholder Values

There are a variety of approaches for starting a dialogue with stakeholders about what they value. We typically begin with facilitated sessions such as focus groups for each major stakeholder segment. These sessions combine education, discussion, and initial surveying of the invited participants. Since it is probably not feasible to involve every physician and every hospital administrator in focus group sessions, your next step is to understand and consolidate the information from these groups and then validate it with an online survey of the broader stakeholder community. This way you not only gain additional insight into the stakeholders, but you involve a larger portion of your community. Figure 6-2 suggests some steps to consider as you begin a dialogue with your stakeholders.

> The Business Plan describes—in detail—*how* you will accomplish your objectives.

At the end of this process, after you have analyzed the results, you will have a clear understanding of what your stakeholders value about HIE, which services they view as important, and the priority in which your stakeholders believe they should be introduced. Interestingly, these typically differ by region, sometimes widely.

THE BUSINESS PLAN

In this section, we focus on two key components of the Business Plan—defining your services and developing your Financial Plan. Initially your business plan activities will resemble a high-level project plan, but as you move into the operation stage, the Business Plan will consist of both project and operational activities.

The Business Plan can be useful in communicating with those individuals and organizations from which you will seek funding and support. It should be developed with an eye toward how you will bring your HIE to the point of operation and your approach to sustainability. The Business Plan sometimes is also referred to as the Operational Plan.

Principles of a Solid Business Plan

According to John Kansky, Vice President, Business Development, Indiana Health Information Exchange (IHIE), there are seven principles upon which IHIE based their Business Plan and from which they make their business decisions. Kansky notes, "Our HIE is a not-for-profit entity. Our mission is to securely provide health information exchange services that improve healthcare quality, safety, and efficiency. These services must provide short-term and long-term value to the entire healthcare community. We don't create a service unless it will break-even in less than two years."

Kansky continues, "Based on the experience of six years of operation and an ongoing history of service development, launch, and support, IHIE bases its sustainability plans on seven basic principles. We believe these principles are key to our health information exchange being a self-sustaining endeavor." Figure 6-3 lists the seven Business Plan principles developed by IHIE.

Components of a Business Plan

The following section describes the components of a good Business Plan. It also explains the key activities you need to undertake to ensure that the plan you develop accurately reflects your strategic plan, moves you closer to fulfilling your mission and achieving your objectives, and puts you on the path to success and sustainability.

Principle 1:	Treat the HIE as a business.
Principle 2:	Leverage high-cost, high-value assets.
Principle 3:	Do not create loss leaders.
Principle 4:	Stay independent and locally sustainable.
Principle 5:	Look for areas where you can have a natural monopoly.
Principle 6:	Pay attention to the need for scale.
Principle 7:	Avoid grants for operational costs.

Figure 6-3: Business Plan Principles Developed by IHIE

1. Executive Summary
2. Organization Description
3. Services to Be Provided
4. Operations Plan
5. Management Plan
6. Financial Plan

Figure 6-4: Components of a Business Plan

Most Business Plans include several components. These components may be called by different names, but their basic purposes are the same. Figure 6-4 provides a high-level list of the Business Plan components we recommend. In this section, we focus on discussions of two of these components: (1) Services to Be Provided [item 3]; and (2) the Financial Plan [item 6]. Other sections of the plan are covered in different sections of this book. The Organization Description and Management Plan [items 2 and 5] are covered in Chapter 4, *Establish a Formal Organizational Governance Structure*, on governance. The initial Operations Plan is covered in Chapter 9, *Becoming Operational*. At the end of this chapter, we provide additional resources including references to actual business plans from operating HIEs.

The work on the Business Plan begins while you are completing your Strategic Plan. In fact, the information generated during your strategic planning process will be the basis for much of your Business Plan. At first, your efforts may be quite informal, but you should quickly migrate from an informal approach to a more formal process that will produce a solid, well thought-out Business Plan.

Defining Your Service Offerings Based upon What Your Stakeholders Value

As mentioned earlier, once you have determined what services your stakeholders value—by engaging them in dialogues—and their perspective of the importance and priority of those services, you are ready to define your initial service offerings. Figure 6-5 lists examples of services we have found that many HIEs provide today, and potential services that could be offered in the future. We have compiled this list through research and by listening to the stakeholders in our various clients' communities. It is provided here to help you generate ideas for the services that your HIE could offer. No single HIE provides all of these services today. Remember, though, that while it is important to understand leading practices and the experience of others, do not let these constrain you. You need to determine what is appropriate for your community.

As part of your initial suite of services, you may want to consider offering administrative services, as well as clinical services. Along with the requirements for clinical services—such as electronic prescribing and refill requests, electronic clinical laboratory ordering and results delivery, electronic public health reporting (i.e., immunizations, notifiable laboratory results), prescription fill status and/or medication fill history, and clinical summary exchange for care coordination and patient engagement—the State HIE Cooperative Agreement Program, which is funding each state's HIE development

Commonly Seen
- Allergies list
- Appointment scheduling
- Claim status inquiry
- Claims submission and response
- Clinical documentation
- Connectivity to personal health records
- Current medical diagnoses
- Current medication list
- Document transfer
- Electronic clinical laboratory ordering
- Electronic notification of claims adjudication results
- Electronic prescribing and refill requests
- Eligibility inquiry and response
- Emergency department episode information
- Immunization registry information
- Inpatient discharge summaries
- Medical record
- Outpatient episode information
- Patient name, demographics, payer, etc.
- Personal health and family history
- Prescription fill history
- Prescription fill status
- Public health reporting
- Quality performance reporting
- Results delivery
- Supply de-identified data for research

Potential or Less Common
- Clinical alerts to providers
- Credentialing information
- Disease management/registry access
- Electronic remittance advice
- Living wills
- Pay-for-performance benchmarks
- Physician contact database
- Quality performance measurement

Figure 6-5: Potential HIE Service Offerings

efforts, contains administrative requirements: electronic eligibility, electronic claims transactions, and quality reporting.

Consider partnering with organizations that already provide services you may want to incorporate into your HIE, such as integrated payment eligibility, claims submission, electronic or real-time remittance, and lab results. Many of these services can be offered through partnerships with other organizations.

Additional services you may want to consider include a provider credentials database, provider contact information, providing a central point for response to patients' requests for electronic versions of their records, and assisting providers with documenting and reporting quality metrics that are required for Meaningful Use incentives and other reporting. The potential services you can provide are limited only by your stakeholders' wants and needs—and your creativity.

Today, there are more opportunities than ever to be creative in developing your services. Many of the incentives for the Meaningful Use of EHRs (see Chapter 1, *The HIE Landscape*, for more information on the meaningful use incentives), relate directly to the sharing of health information and healthcare quality improvements. Use the changes in the healthcare environment to create new services that will be in demand as the healthcare system changes. Your services, and success, should be limited only by your community's desire to improve the quality of healthcare.

The initial services you define, and the costs associated with them, are the foundation for your base revenue model. This list of initial services will also be used by your technology workgroup to determine the functional requirements for the technology that you will need to support and enable your HIE. Expect the management of this list to be an iterative process. Not every desired service can be delivered on day one, but if your stakeholders know you have concrete plans to meet their needs, they are more likely to stay engaged and help you. Documenting and communicating the services you will provide, and the time frame in which they will be rolled out, will help to keep your stakeholders engaged in your efforts.

Figure 6-6 provides key steps you can take to define your services—based on your stakeholders' wants and needs.

Financial Plan

The Financial Plan is a reflection, and cost summary, of the decisions you have made for the business. Within the Financial Plan is your initial, or pro forma, budget. This early budget includes your estimated start-up costs, estimated ongoing operational costs, and anticipated revenue.

The pro forma budget is based upon a set of assumptions. These are assumptions that you have made about the services you will provide, the fees you can charge for those services, the type and amount of resources that you will need to build and support the organization, any potential funding you may receive in addition to your fees, and other components included in your Business Plan. Since the costs of many of your formation efforts will not be known at this point—and your future fee structure will be unproven—developing the initial budget is an exercise in a series of ever-closer approximations.

One of the largest cost categories in the initial budget is often related to the costs associated with technology. A large portion of your budget will be allocated to technology—both for start-up and for your ongoing operations. Even though it is much too early, at this point, to select a technology vendor, you need to have a high-level estimate of the potential costs you will incur. Use your Technical & Security workgroup to help

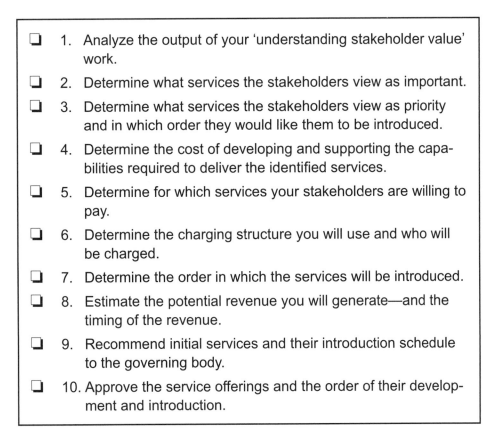

❏   1. Analyze the output of your 'understanding stakeholder value' work.

❏   2. Determine what services the stakeholders view as important.

❏   3. Determine what services the stakeholders view as priority and in which order they would like them to be introduced.

❏   4. Determine the cost of developing and supporting the capabilities required to deliver the identified services.

❏   5. Determine for which services your stakeholders are willing to pay.

❏   6. Determine the charging structure you will use and who will be charged.

❏   7. Determine the order in which the services will be introduced.

❏   8. Estimate the potential revenue you will generate—and the timing of the revenue.

❏   9. Recommend initial services and their introduction schedule to the governing body.

❏   10. Approve the service offerings and the order of their development and introduction.

Figure 6-6: Checklist—Defining Initial Services

provide those estimates. Be sure to communicate to the workgroup that you are only looking for ballpark estimates. You do not want to convey any expectation that they need to gather vendor-specific pricing at this time. Do not be seduced into a premature technology vendor selection when you are only looking for cost estimates. At this point, you do not have a good enough idea of what you need from technology to commit to any specific technology or vendor.

While each HIE budget is unique to the organization, there are categories that are common to most budgets. Figure 6-7 provides example budget categories for you to consider as you build your own budget.

• Building and equipment purchase or lease
• Professional services (legal, consulting)
• Staff salaries
• Software product costs or licensing fees
• Hosting/infrastructure (if applicable)
• Internal staff training & expenses
• Project team tools/software
• Depreciation
• Income/revenue

Figure 6-7: Budget Categories

HIE REVENUE MODELS AND SUSTAINABILITY

The critical objective of attaining long-term financial sustainability is common to all HIEs. Successful HIEs realize that one-time, state-level subsidies and the availability of federal funds associated with HITECH stimulus efforts will not sustain them. We are also seeing that, when it comes to long-term financial sustainability, one proven business model that is appropriate to all HIEs simply does not exist.

In this section, we discuss some potential revenue models and charging approaches for you to consider as you build your Financial Plan. We discuss five models we have seen in use, and we also provide innovative, future approaches for you to consider. In all likelihood, the revenue model you choose will be a combination of the features of two of more of these models. The models we discuss in this section are:

- Membership model
- Transaction Fee model
- Subscription model
- Tax-based model
- Innovative/Future approach
- Supplementary Funding approach

Membership Model

In the pure membership model, HIEs charge a set rate for organizations that want to participate in the exchange. These membership fees are often tiered and are typically based on the size of the organization, their expected resource consumption, or other factors, but every organization is required to join as a member and pay a fee if they want to participate.

An advantage of this model is that it provides predictability to the HIE's revenue stream. Since the memberships generally require a minimum commitment of one year or more, the HIE can rely on that income for a specified period.

One drawback to this model can be that when organizations are members of an HIE, they might have certain expectations. They may believe that since they are members, they are entitled to have a say in how the organization operates or be able to approve new members requesting participation. They may expect to have voting rights and play an active role in decision making. You will need to address these expectations up front and determine if they are compatible with your chosen governance model.

Transaction Fee Model

The transaction fee model is one of the more common HIE revenue models we see today. In the transaction fee model, participants pay a fee for transactions that utilize the HIE. This is a model that can be particularly appealing to the start-up organization as the method for demonstrating a return on investment to stakeholders can be relatively straightforward. For instance, in results delivery, if the electronic transaction process replaces a previous manual or paper model, the costs of the electronic model are generally substantially less than with the current paper-based model.

Another advantage to this revenue model is that there is little up-front financial risk for those participants who want to try out the HIE—since they pay only for the

Example:

In the paper world, labs incur significant costs in delivering their results to individual providers. While those costs may be hidden, they are real costs. The following are some of the hidden costs:

- Staff costs for preparing the paper-based lab results for delivery—sending and resending—the delivery may incur postage, courier, or other delivery costs.
- Staff resources to handle phone calls from providers who need the results before the paper is delivered or who just can't find the paper results that were previously sent.
- The costs of paper and toner or ink cartridges to print the lab results at the provider organization that receives the results.
- The cost in the case of some labs to purchase and provide the fax machines used in the providers' offices as a way to ensure the timely delivery of results.

Once these current—and mostly hidden—costs are identified, the HIE can show that by sending results electronically through the HIE, the costs to the lab for providing results could be significantly reduced. For example, several HIEs have shown that they can deliver results for less than $0.20 per transaction. Compare this cost to the average cost for other delivery methods, which can average more than $0.75 per transaction.

transactions that go through the HIE. This allows them a chance to "get their feet wet" and understand what this is all about before making a larger financial commitment. It also allows them to scale-up their use of the HIE at their own pace—all while producing revenue for the HIE and potential cost savings to the provider.

On the downside, however, we see that some of the more mature HIEs have found that when participants are charged a fee for every transaction, they tend to be less willing to experiment with using the HIE. They may be reluctant to use the HIE's services or try new ideas if they know they will be charged for each transaction.

The transaction model, with its lack of a requirement for a long-term commitment, can lead to an unpredictable revenue stream for the HIE. In addition, you also need to define what constitutes a transaction and define who is charged, and for what. For instance, what do you mean by "transaction"? Do you charge for a request for data? Do you also charge for the transaction that responds to that request? Who should be charged—the requester, the sender, or both? How do you charge if not all of the data are available in a single response? Do you charge for multiple requests or responses? It is not as straightforward as you might initially think, but, by understanding your stakeholders, the questions are answerable.

Another consideration is that as HIEs mature, they begin to find that some of the hospital CFOs or reference lab organizations who were initially very supportive of the transaction fee model because it saved them money are now rethinking their position—not because they are dissatisfied with the HIE but because their costs for transmitting lab results are now very visible; these costs become targets for reduction. The thought goes something like this, "I spend X dollars sending lab results through the HIE every month. I need to show I'm cutting costs. I will just send fewer transactions through the HIE." Instead, they revert back to paper, for which the costs are not so visible. Perhaps this is not the most appropriate or reasonable approach, but it is a reality for at least some of the HIEs with whom we have worked.

We mention this last scenario, not to discourage you from using the transaction fee model—it is a viable model. We mention it to emphasize that you are in a fluid environment and need to constantly be aware of changes in your stakeholders' perspectives and be ready to respond to them.

Subscription Model

In the subscription model, the HIE packages its services into service offerings and provides them—individually or in packages—on a subscription basis to the users of the HIE. We are beginning to see this in some of the more mature HIEs.

Generally, there are multiple types of service offerings available, and participants select the offerings that best meet their needs. Typically, we see where a basic package of services is provided for a set fee; then each participant or organization may add any (currently offered) additional service(s) they desire for an additional fee. Once the participants subscribe to a service, they usually receive unlimited access to the services contained in their subscription.

One advantage to this model is that managing the subscription service can be readily automated, based on the access allowed within the service. Another advantage we are seeing is that participants may be more inclined to increase their use of the HIE, as increased transactions will not directly result in increased fees. We see this as a very customer-focused approach to providing services, since each of the participants can design (to a point) their services packages to meet their individual needs.

The subscription model is advantageous to the HIE as well, since it is usually renewed annually. This provides a predictable revenue stream. Subscription fees can be tiered, based upon the anticipated resource consumption of the participant or the size of the subscribing organization. Tiered pricing provides the appearance of parity in charging, since the participants pay only for the service(s) and service level(s) they select.

Defining and developing services to be charged on a subscription basis compels the HIE to clearly understand the costs for developing and providing each particular service. With clarity of your costs, you can price your component services independently, and this provides you the flexibility to determine, on a per-service basis, the amount of revenue you need to obtain to support that particular service. This approach also helps you build services incrementally when there is a demand.

However, you need to realize that with a subscription service model, as in all models, participants will expect a certain minimum service level. When providing services individually, or ala carte, the consumers of those services will logically begin to associate different costs and values to each of the services. So, for each of your service offerings, you will need to develop service level agreements (SLAs). These define exactly what services will be provided and the constraints (if any) that may be associated with each of the services, such as hours of operation, delivery speed, support, etc. These SLAs will help manage both participant expectations and your obligations for each of your different service offerings. The subscription model requires that you have the processes and resources available to define, document, and consistently meet your SLAs. This requirement could also influence your approach to the technology needed for this model.

Tax-Based Model

Another model that we've seen used is the tax-based model. Some states, such as Vermont, currently levy a tax on every health insurance claims transaction processed in the state. The revenue generated by that tax is then used to support the single, statewide HIE.

An advantage to this funding model is that it can be a predictable and (hopefully) secure revenue stream. Opponents to this model argue that a tax-funded HIE may drive the private sector competition away from the HIE marketplace and stymie free market innovation. There is also another concern that, since the state is supporting the HIE, the state government may demand more of a role in running the HIE than is palatable to the general population. In addition, a state must have a certain level of control over the processing of claims to enact this type of model. As we have said many times, the HIE needs to be sensitive to the culture and norms of the region it serves.

Innovative and Future Funding Approaches

One forward-thinking, innovative funding approach we are beginning to see with some of the state level HIE efforts involves a broadening of the thinking about their sources of revenue and their approach to financial planning. Some states (and HIEs) are working on models that include the Medical Home concept or the Accountable Care Organization approach that incorporates quality improvement efforts to both improve quality

Example:

PHIX (Pennsylvania Health Information eXchange), which is managed by the Governor's Office of Health Care Reform, is exploring combining the State HIE with the Medical Home initiative to create an entity that combines the goals of both programs. The thinking is that by using the HIE to provide clinical documents, such as hospital discharge summaries to primary care providers, and having patients contacted by a care manager within 48 hours after their discharge, many unnecessary hospital readmissions could be prevented. According to their information, the PA Health Care Cost Containment Council has identified 20 reportable conditions, which account for $2.5 billion in hospital readmission charges annually! If using HIE to enable better post-discharge patient results reduces even a portion of the costs for readmission, there would be a solid return on investment along with improved quality outcomes.

Other HIEs, such as MedVirginia and Grand Junction Colorado, are looking at similar quality-based improvements as a model for meeting the goals of quality improvement.

and reduce the costs of healthcare. This model is a bit more complex and longer term than those discussed earlier.

This is an interesting approach and one that is closely aligned with the federal initiatives that promote improving the quality of care. It is a longer-term approach and a more complex revenue model than some of the others we previously discussed, but an approach that we definitely view as innovative and which we expect to see more of as HIEs mature.

Supplementary Funding

There are some additional approaches for funding that you may want to consider as a supplement to your ongoing revenue stream. Grants and fundraising projects can be excellent sources of funding for capital projects, research projects, and even for extending your capabilities. However, we recommend that you not rely on grants or discreet fundraising efforts for your long-term sustainability. That approach simply will not work. However, such efforts can be a good resource to help you grow your HIE business.

Look for other successful capital fundraising campaigns that have been conducted in your community as potential models for your own fundraising efforts. Search and apply for federal, state, local, and organizational grants that can provide the funding for you to develop new organizational capabilities or to offer additional, needed services. Figure 6-8 lists some of the activities you may want to consider as you look to secure additional funding.

Finding Help to Raise Supplementary Funding

It is important to involve people who are knowledgeable in fundraising for non-profit organizations. Consider engaging someone who understands how to conduct a fundraising campaign. Potential resources may be other community not-for-profit organi-

---

❑   1. Research potential funding sources.

❑   2. Determine appropriate activities/outcomes for which the funding will be used, and focus your funding "campaign" on these areas.

❑   3. Identify appropriate funding sources.

❑   4. Communicate the HIE's need for funding.

❑   5. Discuss with potential funding sources the value they should expect to receive from providing funds.

❑   6. Create the business case for the funding request.

❑   7. Develop the application for funding source(s).

❑   8. Receive notice of funding.

Figure 6-8: Checklist—Finding Funding Sources

zations, community development organizations, universities, and even small business assistance groups.

You may also want to consider involving someone with knowledge of grant resources who is experienced in writing grant proposals. Your local colleges or universities can be good resources for these skills.

WHOM TO INVOLVE IN BUILDING THE BUSINESS PLAN

You will need to involve people knowledgeable in the multiple aspects of building a Business Plan. Many of these folks are probably already members of your various workgroups or committees. Ensure that each workgroup contributes their recommendations to the Business Plan.

We recommend that you also engage an individual or firm that is familiar with the HIE environment. They can point you to appropriate resources and connect you with other HIEs that can assist you and can provide you with information gleaned from their own experiences.

Many excellent examples of Business Plans can be found online. In addition, the State HIE Cooperative Agreement Program also requires that each state submit their overall HIE business (operations) plan. Most of these are publically available and can serve as a good reference. We list several in the resource section at the end of this chapter. Figure 6-9 summarizes the business plan development roadmap.

❑ 1. Review your vision, mission, objectives, strategies, and initiatives to ensure that they are understood by all involved in your organization.

❑ 2. Review Business Plans from your state and other HIEs that are in areas with similar geographic and demographic characteristics.

❑ 3. Address the barriers identified during your community assessment efforts.

❑ 4. Determine the various risks to your developing HIE and define and document your risk mitigation plans.

❑ 5. Define your initial services and the order in which they will be introduced.

❑ 6. Develop your Financial Plan.

❑ 7. Compile the various plan components into a consolidated Business Plan document.

❑ 8. Circulate the Business Plan broadly for review, comment, and buy-in.

❑ 9. Incorporate comments as appropriate.

❑ 10. Present the Business Plan to the board for approval.

Figure 6-9: Checklist—Building a Business Plan

As stated previously, creating your Business Plan requires a multi-faceted approach. You will need to involve a diverse group of people with a variety of skill sets. Engage people knowledgeable in all aspects of building a Business Plan, as well as people knowledgeable about HIEs.

As you develop your funding models, you undoubtedly will examine multiple potential funding streams. You may want to start with transaction fees because it is an approach that is relatively straightforward and will provide some initial revenue as you build your HIE. Once your HIE is operational, you will have even better insight into what your stakeholders value. Help them learn how to use the HIE. Stay connected with them and solicit their feedback—and they will tell you what additional services they need.

CHAPTER SUMMARY

In this chapter, we discussed creating your initial Business Plan and the importance of having a continuing dialogue with your stakeholders to both understand what they value and to ensure their ongoing participation.

We discussed engaging your stakeholders directly to determine what services you should offer and in what order they should be offered.

The Business Plan describes in detail how you will achieve your mission and run your organization. We focused on two key components of the Business Plan: (1) determining the services you will provide; and (2) developing your Financial Plan. We provided examples of revenue models for you to consider as you build your Financial Plan.

When you complete the activities in this chapter, you will have:

- An appreciation of the importance of dialoguing with your stakeholders to understand what they value and how what they value can be used to design your services;
- Defined an initial set of service offerings;
- Determined the type of revenue model(s) you will initially pursue; and
- An initial Business Plan.

CASE STUDIES
Delaware Health Information Network (DHIN)

Gina Bianco Perez, Executive Director, Delaware Health Information Network

DHIN's business model was built in two phases. During Phase 1, they built the infrastructure, network, functions and features, and the user base. In Phase 1, they received capital funds from the state and a dollar-for-dollar match on the private side, which is based on a transaction-based fee structure. DHIN is preparing to embark on Phase 2, which is the operational phase, where all of the base functionality has been implemented and the majority of healthcare providers are using the system. The sustainability model will move from one of capital funding to one of a fee-based model that is related to benefit derived from the system.

Indiana Health Information Exchange (IHIE)

John Kansky, Vice President, Indiana Health Information Exchange

IHIE is a not-for-profit entity whose mission is to securely provide health information exchange services that improve healthcare quality, safety, and efficiency. These services must provide short-term and long-term value to the entire healthcare community. Kansky notes, "We don't create a service unless it will break-even in less than two years."

The current revenue model is based on transaction fees for its results delivery service. For other services, IHIE charges participant fees.

Based on the experience of six years of operation and an ongoing history of service development, launch, and support, IHIE bases its sustainability plans on seven basic principles, which they believe are key to health information exchange being a self-sustaining endeavor. These principles are listed in Figure 6-3.

Kansky recommends the following straightforward process to developing a revenue model:

1. Start with something relatively easy to deliver, such as results delivery. This will build the revenue stream for maintaining the infrastructure and provide a mechanism to standardize clinical information across providers. There is a basic return on investment (ROI) that is easy for potential customers to understand. The ROI is based on decreasing the costs associated with returning results to providers. For example, hospitals currently spend large amounts to send paper results—by mail, fax, or courier. An HIE can help these organizations identify and quantify these [paper-related] costs and then offer to provide the service at a significant reduction, using electronic delivery and "one-stop sending."

2. A solid revenue stream and clinical information standardization enables an HIE to build more sophisticated services such as clinical repository services to provide, for example, a comprehensive, 'virtual' patient record at the point of care.

3. Once these infrastructure capabilities are in place, along with a revenue stream, an HIE can provide other value-added services such as quality monitoring and reporting.

Kansky also identifies several factors that he believes are critical as you consider which services to include in your business model.

1. The market has to be a big enough pool of potential customers who will be interested in a service to make it sustainable.

2. The ROI must be easy for a CFO to understand and agree to support. Just doing something for the good of society will not necessarily convince CFOs to recommend that their organizations participate.

3. Your HIE must provide excellent execution of the services you deliver. You cannot be second rate at delivery.

4. The services you select should have fixed infrastructure costs and should allow you to reuse your resources.

For example, if your infrastructure costs $1.00 to run, offer a variety of services at 60 cents, 30 cents, and 10 cents versus offering only one service for $1.00.

Offer a good mix of services that interest several types of stakeholders.

Lessons Learned

IHIE has been in business long enough that their customers have matured in their approach to and use of their services. A key lesson learned is that the HIE organization must always be sensitive to their stakeholders' needs. As the HIE's stakeholders mature in their use of HIE services, their needs and perspectives on the revenue model may also change. As a result of the constant dialogue with their stakeholders, IHIE is now considering additional sources of revenue to be introduced over the next several years. The plan is to keep the demand for their services at a sustainable level.

HealthBridge

Trudi Matthews, Director Policy and Public Relations, HealthBridge

HealthBridge can trace its beginnings to an unsuccessful CHIN effort in the 1990s. The major employers in the region were very interested in centralizing claims information to drive down costs in the region. While the providers were not in favor of this approach, the general threat of this happening without their input solidified the provider community's commitment to use technology and collaboration to improve healthcare in the Greater Cincinnati community.

HealthBridge began with two health plans and five health systems. This group of stakeholders became the founders of HealthBridge. These stakeholders were serious about forming an HIE as demonstrated by the fact that each of these founders committed to provide loans of $250,000—a total of $1.75 million—to launch the effort. In return, they were given a board seat on the new organization. This set up a unique motivation for the organization to be successful in that the repayment of the loans to the founders was dependent upon the organization's success. In other words, they had a responsibility to pay themselves back. HealthBridge, since early 2003, has been profitable, earning 5%–8% over expenses each year.

The first service offered by the new organization was a combined portal/gateway into inpatient information systems. This provided remote access to physicians.

The success of the portal led to the next step. Clinical messaging was deployed in 2000 with one hospital and grew over time to include more hospitals and labs and more types of clinical information. The health systems agreed to outsource their information and pay monthly subscription fees to HealthBridge to host the portal and messaging. Fees were based on the size of the organization.

Over time, HealthBridge added additional hospitals to that service to the point where HealthBridge became the outsourced means for all large healthcare systems to deliver results to the community.

As their revenue increased from providing services to an expanding list of providers, Health Bridge gained momentum. In 2004–2005, as more providers adopted EHRs, HealthBridge moved to provide a single interface to deliver lab results into an EHR. The majority of physicians who have EHRs pay a small fee for this service. Physicians are willing to pay this fee because they see value in dealing with only a single interface for receiving results. They find this much easier than needing to interface with multiple disparate systems. For the CIOs of hospitals, this single interface provides value in that they now send their results to one system—and that system normalizes the results for the many disparate EHR systems receiving the results—and sends them to the appropriate recipients.

While the majority of revenue for HealthBridge comes from results delivery, they have diversified into other premium service areas as well. These additional services include transcription, billing, e-prescribing, registry, and assisting with EHR adoption by providers through its Regional Extension Center.

As an experienced, successful HIE, HealthBridge offers the following insights:

- Start with a few participants and services and build adoption.
- Run a pilot, make sure it works well, and ensure that you are able to scale the system.
- Start with small, affordable steps and build capacity from there.

HealthBridge credits listening to their customers very closely as a key to their success. They work with their stakeholders to identify areas that are common "pain points." They develop service offerings for those areas that can be addressed through the appropriate, collaborative use of technology.

Nebraska Health Information Initiative (NeHII)

Deb Bass, Executive Director, Nebraska Health Information Initiative

The Nebraska Health Information Initiative (NeHII) currently derives its revenue from license fees for the edge servers (they provide) at each organization participating in the HIE. NeHII provides the servers and the associated software for the data providers to connect to the HIE via a Virtual Private Network.

Their fee structure is based on the type and size of the participant:

- Hospitals that are data providers pay a graduated fee based upon bed size. The fees range from $1,500 per month to $12,000 per month based upon their size.
- Labs and pharmacies are charged $2,000 per month for a single-direction connection and $3,000 per month for a bi-directional connection. To entice independent labs to join the HIE, NeHII has made special discount pricing available to the first two independent labs that sign participation agreements.
- NeHII provides physicians with either a Virtual Health Record (VHR) for $20 per month or an EHR with e-prescribing capabilities for $51.66 per month.

The services provided by NeHII include:

- Master Patient Index (MPI)
- Record Locator Service (RLS)
- Medication history
- Prescription fill information
- Allergy notification
- Insurance eligibility
- Transcription reports, including but not limited to:
  - Hospital admission
  - Discharge summaries
  - Operative reports
  - Lab and clinical messaging
- Public health reporting, disease surveillance and immunization registry are in process

RESOURCES

Maryland HIE Strategic and Operational Plan
http://mhcc.maryland.gov/electronichealth/hiestateplan/hit_state_plan_060910.pdf. Accessed October, 2010.

New Mexico HIE Strategic and Operation Plan
http://statehieresources.org/wp-content/uploads/2009/12/NMStateHIEStrategicandOperationalPlanV2.pdf. Accessed October, 2010.

Utah Operational Plan
http://health.utah.gov/phi/ehealth/UT_HIE_OperationalPlan_March2010.pdf. Accessed October, 2010.

Department of Health & Human Services. Meaningful Use. http://healthit.hhs.gov/portal/server.pt?open=512&objID=1325&parentname=CommunityPage&parentid=1&mode=2. Accessed November, 2009.

Minnesota Health Information Exchange. MN HIE Services. http://www.mnhie.org/services.html. Accessed November, 2009.

Indiana University & the Regenstrief Institute. HIE Services Available.
http://www.regenstrief.org/medinformatics/inpc/hie-services-available/Summary%20Indiana%20HIE%20Services.pdf. Accessed November, 2009.

California Regional Health Information Organization. CalRHIO Services.
http://www.calrhio.org/?cridx=421. Accessed November, 2009.

Health Unity. RHIO Services Node.
http://www.healthunity.com/handbook_rhioservicesnode.aspx. Accessed November, 2009.

McDonald CJ, Overhage JM, Barnes M, Schadow G, Blevins L, Dexter PR, Mamlin B; INPC Management Committee. The Indiana Network for Patient Care: A Working Local Health Information Infrastructure. An Example of a Working Infrastructure Collaboration that Links Data from Five Health Systems and Hundreds of Millions of Entries. *Health Affairs*. 2005; 24(5):1214-1220. http://www.ncbi.nlm.nih.gov/sites/entrez?Db=pubmed&Cmd=ShowDetailView&TermToSearch=16162565. Accessed April, 2010.

California State Rural Health Association (CSRHA). Capital Campaign Toolkit.
http://www.csrha.org/usda/capital_campaign_toolkit_csrha08.pdf. Accessed November, 2009.

McNamara C. Overview of Nonprofit Fundraising Sources and Approaches. 1997.
http://managementhelp.org/fndrsng/np_raise/fndraise.htm. Accessed November, 2009.

Department of Health & Human Services. Tips for Writing Grant Proposals.
http://www.hhs.gov/grantsnet/AppTips.htm. Accessed November, 2009.

Center for Information Technology Leadership (CITL). *The Value of Healthcare Information Exchange and Interoperability*. Wellesley, MA: CITL; 2004. http://www.citl.org/news/Interop_Release_FINAL.pdf. Accessed April, 2010.

Example HIE Business Plans

Delaware Health Information Network Business Plan. Posted November 14, 2009. http://healthit.hhs.gov/portal/server.pt/gateway/PTARGS_0_10731_848175_0_0_18/DHIN%20Business%20Plan_NHIN%20%20Final.pdf. Accessed November, 2009.

IHIE Business Plan. Posted January 12, 2009. http://healthit.hhs.gov/portal/server.pt/gateway/PTARGS_0_10731_848176_0_0_18/Indiana_Business_Plan_NHIN_Final.pdf. Accessed November, 2009.

MedVirginia Strategic Business Plan. Posted November 14, 2008. http://healthit.hhs.gov/portal/server.pt/gateway/PTARGS_0_10731_848177_0_0_18/MedVirginia%20Business%20Plan_NHIN_Final.pdf. Accessed November, 2009.

New York eHealth Collaborative Jurisdiction-Specific Business Plan. Posted November 13, 2009. http://healthit.hhs.gov/portal/server.pt/gateway/PTARGS_0_10731_848179_0_0_18/NYeC%20Business%20Plan_NHIN_Final.pdf. Accessed November, 2009.

New Mexico State HIT Plan.
http://NMHIC.org.

West Virginia Health Information Network Business Plan. Posted November 14, 2008. http://healthit.hhs.gov/portal/server.pt/gateway/PTARGS_0_10731_848180_0_0_18/WVHIN_Business_Plan_NHIN_Final.pdf. Accessed November, 2009.

CHAPTER 7

Protecting Patient Privacy

"Build privacy into your exchange from the very beginning."

Jeff Blair
Director of Health Informatics
LCF Research/New Mexico Health Information Collaborative

INTRODUCTION

Privacy is personal. This chapter is about privacy—not privacy and security. We have intentionally separated privacy from security in this book because we believe that privacy and security are two different things.

Privacy is what you, as a health information organization, are required to protect. Privacy is the *what*. Privacy addresses the rights of patients to have their information protected and kept confidential.

Security, on the other hand is the *how*. It refers to how you enable that protection and consists of the policies, processes, measures, and controls that enable the privacy of patient information to be maintained. We discuss security in more detail in Chapter 8, *The Time for Technology*, as much of security relates to—and is implemented through—your technology infrastructure.

A great deal has already been written about the subject of privacy. When reviewing that information, it's easy to become confused and even overwhelmed. It may seem that there are as many different opinions and points of view on the subject as there are articles. While the discussion of privacy may tend to cause confusion, we believe the discussion is healthy because ensuring patient privacy is an important topic and one that is critical to your success. While any initial confusion you have about privacy won't last long, your concern about privacy should continue forever.

In this chapter we describe the key points relating to privacy that you need to be aware of and should take into consideration as you continue on your journey of building a successful, sustainable, and secure HIE for your community.

Many of your organization's policies will be a reflection of its obligations under federal and state laws and regulations that relate to the expectation of privacy of personal health information. These regulations serve as the floor for the various levels of privacy protection that you must implement.

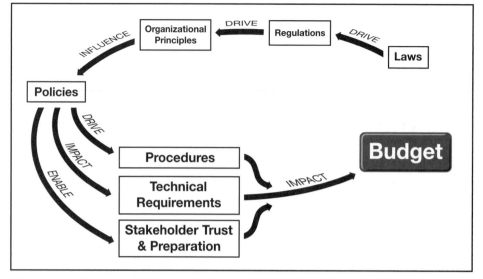

Figure 7-1: Drivers of Privacy Policies. © 2009 Mosaica Partners, LLC. Used by permission.

The subject of privacy, as it relates to HIE, is evolving and will continue to evolve for the foreseeable future. This chapter provides a guide to developing your privacy policies and provides a rich list of resources to assist you. Remember, this is an area that requires you to be in strict compliance with both federal and state laws and regulations. You should definitely seek legal advice as you develop and finalize your privacy policies. As consultants and authors, we do not purport to offer either legal advice or opinion. That can only be provided by your legal advisor.

The protection of personal health information from exposure to inappropriate disclosure, access, or modification—whether accidental or intentional—is mandated under federal and state law. However, perhaps even more significant, is that the guarantee of the privacy of personal health information is paramount to any HIE's ability to garner and maintain trust in the organization. A critical success factor for any HIE is the ability for all of its participants and patients to trust that the HIE (1) limits the use of their personal health information; (2) makes their information available only to permitted recipients; and (3) has taken the necessary steps to ensure the confidentiality, integrity, and quality of their health information.

The need to ensure privacy will drive and impact almost every area of your planning. You will use your privacy policies as the basis for your operational policies and procedures (see Figure 7-1). Your privacy policies are the framework upon which you build your organization's security infrastructure (administrative, physical, and technical), and they must be taken into consideration as you plan and develop your various service offerings. As Ted Kremer, Executive Director of the Rochester, NY RHIO, comments, "RHIOs really need to think about their privacy model up front."

THE BACKGROUND OF PRIVACY REQUIREMENTS

It is important that you begin with a high-level understanding of the relevant privacy laws and regulations and how they relate to your HIE. Most of the laws and regulations we list in the following section deal with a person's right to privacy related to his or her personal health information. The privacy laws address access to, and the use and disclosure of, a person's health information, as well as some of the penalties for misuse of that information. To put the current landscape of patient privacy protection in context, we expand upon the information from Chapter 1, *The HIE Landscape*, with a short discussion on the background of privacy law in the U.S.

Federal Laws Guiding Adoption and Use of HIT/HIE

The Health Insurance Portability and Accountability Act (HIPAA), which became federal law in 1996, may be one of the most widely recognized statutes regarding privacy and security of electronic information. However, the U.S. laws and principles pertaining to the protection of personal information stored electronically go back more than 30 years.

Fair Information Practices Principles

The privacy laws and regulations adopted in the U.S. in the last few decades are based upon a commonly accepted set of fair information practices. The earliest public documentation of this concept was published in 1973 in the report "Records, Computers and the Rights of Citizens,"[1] which introduced Fair Information Practices Principles[2] (FIPPs). These principles created a code of fair information practices that addressed the collection, maintenance, use, and dissemination of personal information by federal executive branch agencies. The four FIPPs are:

1. **Notice:** There must be no personal data record-keeping systems whose very existence is secret.
   a. Data collectors must disclose their data collection.
   b. The existence and purpose of record-keeping systems must be known to the individuals whose data is contained therein.
2. **Choice:** There must be a way for a person to find out what personal information is contained in a record and how it may be used.
   a. There must be a way for a person to prevent personal information that was obtained for one purpose from being used or made available for other purposes without the person's consent.
   b. Data subjects should have the right to opt out of uses and disclosures of their data.
   c. Information must be (1) collected only with the knowledge and implicit or explicit permission of the subject; (2) used only in ways relevant to the purpose for which the data was collected; and (3) disclosed only with permission of the subject or in accordance with overriding legal authority (such as a public health law that requires reporting of a serious contagious disease).
3. **Access:** There must be a way for a person to correct or amend a record of identifiable personal information.
   a. Data subjects should be able to view their information and have it corrected if necessary.
   b. Individuals must have the right to see records of personal information and to assure the quality of that information.

4. **Security:** Any organization creating, maintaining, using, or disseminating records of identifiable personal data must assure the reliability of the data for their intended use and must take precautions to prevent misuses of the data.
   a. Reasonable safeguards must be in place to protect the confidentiality, integrity, and availability of information.

The application of FIPPs to HIE is discussed and refined in the Markle Foundation's "Connecting for Health: Common Framework."[3]

Privacy Act of 1974

The Privacy Act of 1974, 5 U.S.C. § 552a, establishes a code of fair information practices that governs the collection, maintenance, use, and dissemination of personally identifiable information about individuals that is maintained in systems of records by federal agencies.[4] This act prevents federal agencies from disclosing any record, which is contained in a system of records, without the prior written consent of the individual whose information is contained in the record.

The Privacy Act of 1974 and its implementing regulations:
1. Prohibits the *disclosure* of personally identifiable information maintained by agencies in a system of records without the consent of the subject individual, subject to twelve codified exceptions.
2. Grants individuals increased rights of *access* to agency records maintained on them.
3. Grants individuals the right to seek *amendment* of agency records that are maintained on them upon showing that the records are not accurate, relevant, timely, or complete.
4. Establishes a code of *fair information practices* that requires agencies to comply with statutory norms for the collection, maintenance, and dissemination of records.

Health Insurance Portability and Accountability Act of 1996

In the 1990s, the increasing use of health IT created a focus on the need to standardize the technical aspects of the exchange of personal health information. Along with standardization arose the issue of protecting personal health information from disclosure or misuse. This prompted legislative action. The Health Insurance Portability and Accountability Act[5]—commonly referred to as HIPAA—became federal law in 1996 and may be one of the most widely recognized statutes regarding the privacy and security of electronic information. Grounded by the FIPPs, HIPAA outlined the basic elements of a series of healthcare regulations.

The Administrative Simplification provisions of HIPAA, Title II,[6] and the regulations promulgated under it address the "Security standards for the protection of electronic health information" and "Privacy of identifiable health information." These provisions address in detail the security and privacy of electronic health data and require compliance with a comprehensive set of requirements to assure the security of information architectures. These rules state that *covered entities*, which include payers, providers, and claims clearinghouses, must follow the guidelines shown in Figure 7-2.

- Ensure the confidentiality, integrity, and availability of all electronic protected health information the covered entity creates, receives, maintains, or transmits.
- Protect against any reasonable anticipated threats or hazards to the security or integrity of such information.
- Protect against any reasonable anticipated use or disclosure of such information that are not permitted or required under the law.
- Ensure compliance by its workforce.

Figure 7-2: Adapted from HIPAA Title II Rules

HIPAA Title II specifically states that covered entities must implement administrative, physical, and technical safeguards for protecting electronic health information. The act also creates a privacy right with respect to personally identifiable health information and sets forth requirements related to the use and disclosure of health information, the types of authorization required for release of that information, and when an individual has the opportunity to approve or object to its release. Significantly, HIPAA allows the exchange of information without patient authorization in the broad areas of treatment, payment, and healthcare operations.[7]

The act also outlines the rights of an individual and the notification of those rights to the person to request their own health information, how entities must account for disclosures of health information, and the administrative policies and procedures required for implementation of the standards.

In addition to the FIPPs principles (many of which were incorporated into HIPAA), and HIPAA itself, there are other federal laws and regulations of which you must be aware and take into consideration as you develop your privacy policies. Figure 7-3 provides an overview of some of the key laws and regulations. This information has been excerpted from "Summary of Selected Federal Laws and Regulations Addressing Confidentiality, Privacy, and Security."[8]

For a more complete summary of the laws and regulations that address confidentiality, privacy, and security, visit the U.S. Department of Health & Human Services, Privacy and Security Home Page.[9] Examples of additional laws and regulations that may apply include the Federal Trade Commission Act,[10] Gramm Leach Bliley,[11] Sarbanes Oxley,[12] PCI Security Standard,[13] Family Educational Rights and Privacy Act[14] (FERPA), and Employee Retirement Income Security Act (ERISA) of 1974.[15]

HHS Privacy and Security Framework Principles

As part of its ongoing work on the Nationwide Health Information Network, HHS developed the Privacy and Security Framework Principles.[16] These principles, shown in Figure 7-4, establish a consistent approach to address the privacy and security challenges related to electronic health information exchange through a broad, inclusive network.

The goal of these principles is to establish a policy framework for electronic health information exchange to promote the adoption of health information technologies in

Federal Law	Summary
Health Insurance Portability and Accountability Act (HIPAA), Privacy Rule (2000)	Establishes national standards regarding health information privacy. Creates a *federal floor* of health information privacy protection; some more protective state laws remain in force. The Privacy Rule creates certain individual rights in health information, imposes restrictions on uses and disclosures of protected health information, and provides for civil and criminal penalties for violations.
Health Insurance Portability and Accountability Act (HIPAA), Security Rule	Establishes nationally required and addressable security standards. Works in tandem with the HIPAA Privacy Rule and lays out three types of security safeguards required for compliance: administrative, physical, and technical.
HITECH Act Breach Notification Rule (Health & Human Services)	Amends HIPAA to require notification by HIPAA covered entities—upon the discovery of a breach of security. Requires covered entities to provide notice to patients, HHS, and in some cases, the media, following a breach of unsecured protected health information. Also requires business associates to notify covered entities following the discovery of such a breach.

Figure 7-3: Excerpted from "Summary of Selected Federal Laws and Regulations Addressing Confidentiality, Privacy, and Security," Department of Health & Human Services.[8]

Federal Law	Summary
SAMHSA: Confidentiality of Substance Abuse Patient Records	Addresses the confidentiality of substance abuse patient records (alcohol and drug abuse patient records).
	Prohibits the disclosure of substance abuse patient records, and information that identifies an individual as an alcohol or drug abuser, without obtaining the written consent of the individual.
	The regulations establish limited circumstances permitting disclosures without consent for medical emergencies, audit/evaluation activities, and research. Other disclosures without patient consent are permitted with an authorizing court order issued by a court of competent jurisdiction.
Clinical Laboratory Improvement Amendments (CLIA) (1988)	Regulates laboratories conducting testing on human specimens for medical purposes.
	Assures quality standards for all laboratory testing to ensure the accuracy, reliability, and timeliness of patient test results.
	Certified labs may disclose test results or reports only to authorized people, those responsible for using the results (i.e., those treating the patient), and the referring lab in a reference lab scenario; state laws define who is authorized, which may include the patient.
SAMHSA: Confidentiality Provisions for Data Collection and Survey Information	*Requires the consent* of the person or establishment prior to use or release of identifiable information.
	Identifiable information obtained in the course of activities undertaken or supported by SAMHSA pursuant to data collection authorized activities may not be used for any purpose other than the purpose for which it was supplied unless such establishment or person has consented (as determined under regulations of the Secretary) to its use for such other purpose.

Figure 7-3: *Continued*

the U.S. The principles were designed to establish and define the roles of individuals and the responsibilities of those who hold and exchange electronic individually identifiable health information through a network. These principles, which closely follow FIPPs, provide a good foundation upon which to build your organization's privacy principles. For more information, see the HIMSS Privacy & Security Toolkit[17] and the HHS Privacy and Security Toolkit.[18]

- **Individual Access**—Individuals should be provided with a simple and timely means to access and obtain their individually identifiable health information in a readable form and format.
- **Correction**—Individuals should be provided with a timely means to dispute the accuracy or integrity of their individually identifiable health information, and to have erroneous information corrected or to have a dispute documented if their requests are denied.
- **Openness and Transparency**—There should be openness and transparency about policies, procedures, and technologies that directly affect individuals and/or their individually identifiable health information.
- **Individual Choice**—Individuals should be provided a reasonable opportunity and capability to make informed decisions about the collection, use, and disclosure of their individually identifiable health information.
- **Collection, Use, and Disclosure Limitation**—Individually identifiable health information should be collected, used, and/or disclosed only to the extent necessary to accomplish a specified purpose(s) and never to discriminate inappropriately.
- **Data Quality and Integrity**—Persons and entities should take reasonable steps to ensure that individually identifiable health information is complete, accurate, and up to date to the extent necessary for the person's or entity's intended purposes and has not been altered or destroyed in an unauthorized manner.
- **Safeguards**—Individually identifiable health information should be protected with reasonable administrative, technical, and physical safeguards to ensure its confidentiality, integrity, and availability and to prevent unauthorized or inappropriate access, use, or disclosure.
- **Accountability**—These principles should be implemented, and adherence assured, through appropriate monitoring and other means and methods should be in place to report and mitigate non-adherence and breaches.

Figure 7-4: HHS Privacy and Security Framework Principles

PRIVACY IMPLICATIONS ON POLICIES

To ensure that you are fully protecting a person's right to privacy, you must ensure that: (1) any person seeking access to health information has the right to access the data; (2) the person is who he or she claims to be; and (3) the person is permitted access to the data. You must be able to provide, on request of a patient, a list of all accesses to that person's data and ensure that you hold anyone accountable for inappropriate access or use of the data.

While privacy and security are two different areas, there is overlap between them. To help you structure your understanding and approach to privacy policies, we address them in five broad *security*-related categories. We call these the "5 A's of Security," and they are summarized in Figure 7-5.

The following section discusses each of these five components, including key questions you need to answer as you develop your privacy policies in each of the areas. Later, in Chapter 8, *The Time for Technology*, we will discuss these components in more detail from the security perspective.

Authentication

Authentication[19] is the process of proving that a user (or a system) that is requesting access is really who (or what) it claims to be. This is used to protect against the fraudulent use of a system or the fraudulent transmission of information.

Authentication is a core element in protecting the privacy of a patient's information by assuring access only to those who have a right to see it. While authentication of users within an organization may be straightforward, in an HIE environment you need to ensure that those requesting access across multiple institutions, and even patients themselves, are who they claim to be. The remainder of the "5 A's" are based upon this critical component.

Authentication
> Ensuring that individuals logging into the system are who they say they are.

Authorization
> Determining that individuals are allowed to access the HIE.

Access to data
> Determining to which data individuals have access and what actions they are allowed to take relative to that data.

Audit policies
> Ensuring that you can consistently inspect what records have been accessed and by whom.

Accountability
> Determining how you will hold those responsible for security breaches liable.

Figure 7-5: The 5 A's of Security

Questions to address as you develop Authentication policies:
- How will you ensure that the individuals logging into the system are who they say they are?
- How will you accommodate the multiple authentication processes in use at the various participants of your HIE?
- What are your obligations as a HIPAA Business Associate to ensure appropriate authentication of all of the users of your HIE?

Authorization

Authorization determines what rights each person has in the system once access is allowed. Authorization requires that the system can identify the user and relate the user's identification (ID) to the specific areas within the system that the person may be allowed to access. Authorization requires that the user has been registered with, and approved to use, the system. In addition, the system must be aware of who the user is and be able to associate the user ID with specific permissions to access specific types of data.

For example: If '*user ID 12345*' is requesting system access, the system must know that '*user ID 12345*' was approved to use the system and that the system can associate '*user ID 12345*' with specific rights to access specific types of data in the system.

Questions to address as you develop Authorization policies:
- What policies do you need to determine that a person is allowed to access the HIE?
- What policies are required to associate specific user IDs with approved uses of the system?
- What policies will you employ to register users of the system?
- What policies do you need to make sure that users are authorized only to access the parts of the system that are relevant and necessary?

Access to Data

Access to data is a continuation of the authorization process. Once a person has been authenticated and his or her ID has been authorized to connect to the HIE, you must then determine what rights that person has to access the different types of data in the system. Access policies address what information a person may and may not access and what actions the person may perform on the accessed data. Granting access to data may involve different types of allowed actions. Access policies address whether the requester may read (view) the data, modify the data, and/or delete the data. Access to data is generally granted based upon three key components:
- The user's approved level and type of authorization;
- The user's reason to access the data and the types of actions the person may perform; and
- The patient's consent for sharing his or her information.

Many healthcare organizations use a process known as "role-based" access that associates the person's logon ID with the various levels of access and permitted activities—roles. With this approach, each person (represented by a unique user ID) is assigned one or multiple roles. Each role has specifically defined rights of access to, and actions it can perform on, data in the system. We discuss this in more detail in Chapter 8, *The Time for Technology*.

Patient Consent to Access of Data

In providing access to data, it is also important to consider whether patients must consent to access to their data. Under HIPAA, patient consent is not required for a covered entity to use or disclose identifiable health information if it is only used for treatment, payment, or healthcare operations. Broader uses of patient data require specific patient consent. State law may further address the requirement for patient consent for the sharing of information through an HIE. For example, many state laws require patient consent for access to certain types of sensitive health information. A small number of states have laws that require consent for *any* access.

The discussion of patient consent is generally framed around whether a patient has "opted in" to the exchange or "opted out." In some cases, state law regulates the type of approach used. However, since we are in the early stages of addressing privacy and the access to, and the sharing of, electronic health information, many states are still formulating their laws. In this section we briefly discuss the two basic options related to a patient's consent to participating in an HIE—the "Opt-In" model and the "Opt-Out" model. Make sure you understand your own state's requirements.

Patient "Opt-In" Model

In states or HIEs with laws or policies specifying that a patient must "opt-in" to the exchange, a patient's data, by default, are not accessible for exchange unless the patient specifically provides written consent for data to be shared. Generally, this consent is obtained at the time the care provider obtains consent for care and informs the patient of his or her privacy rights.

Opt-in consent may range from a patient opting in to the exchange for all their data, to a point at which the patient is able to specify exactly what data may be shared and with whom it may be shared. How the opt-in approach to patient consent is implemented depends not only on the applicable laws but also on the norms and culture of your community, your policies, and the capabilities of your security tools.

Caution: Complying with a patient's opt-in requests that are data-specific or provider-specific can be a cumbersome process that is technically complex and costly. This is due in part to the need to identify the individual components of the record to determine who may, or may not, have access.

Patient "Opt-Out" Model

In states or HIEs operating under the "Opt-Out" model, a patient's health information is included in the exchange unless he or she specifically requests, in writing, to opt out of the exchange. In this model, all patient information is automatically included in the exchange, and his or her data are available to be shared, within the appropriate authorization and access policies, with all the other participants in the exchange.

As with opt-in, opting out of participating in an HIE is approached differently in different states and regions, based on their stakeholder requirements. For example, HealthInfoNet in Maine,[20] which has an opt-out policy, includes a patient's data in the exchange unless the patient specifically opts out in writing. If a patient opts out of the exchange, that patient's data are blocked from inclusion in the exchange and are not available for sharing.

Questions to address as you develop Access policies:

- What are the applicable laws in your state relating to a patient's consent for participation in the HIE?
- What policies do you need to implement to meet the stakeholder needs and concerns in your community?
- What policies are needed to determine to which data a person has access and what specific actions they are allowed to take relative to those data?
- How will you determine to which data a person has access and what actions they are allowed to take relative to those data?

Break the Glass

There is a lot of discussion, and a variety of opinions, when it comes to the issue of making patient information available through the HIE in an emergency situation. The phrase "break the glass" refers to overriding some of the normal access restrictions to a patient's data in emergency situations. Generally, this occurs when an authorized user needs access to a patient's information in an urgent situation, and the normally required conditions for the patient's consent have not been met or certain requirements for authentication cannot be met in time.

Access under these conditions requires that you understand your relevant state laws. You must have specific policies and procedures in place to ensure that patient confidentiality is maintained, only appropriate access is allowed, the patient is informed of the access, and the appropriate audit trail is maintained.

Questions to address as you develop "break the glass" policies:

- What are the relevant laws in your state relating to access to information in an emergency situation?
- Under what conditions is a provider allowed to use the "break the glass" procedure?
- What is the specific process a provider must follow?
- What types of authorization and follow-up actions are required?
- How is "break the glass" access controlled and monitored?
- Are the data of a patient who has opted out of the exchange still available to providers in an emergency situation?
- How, and when, are patients informed if a "break the glass" situation has occurred?

Audit

HIPAA's Privacy Rule grants individuals the right to be informed about how their personal health information has been used and disclosed. To remain in compliance with current privacy regulations, you need to be able to provide to patients (upon request) information on all accesses to their data that have occurred for other than treatment, payment, and healthcare operations. Under the Health Information Technology for Economic and Clinical Health (HITECH) Act, the scope of the required accounting was expanded to include treatment, payment, operations (TPO) disclosures,[21] and this has been included in the final rule. In addition, you are required to not only track accesses to health data but to also take steps to prevent and detect any breaches.

Audit policies are implemented to ensure that you remain in compliance with your established policies and procedures. Auditing access to data requires that transaction logs be kept and monitored for every data access for every record. The process for detecting misuse can be approached in a couple of ways, both retrospectively and prospectively.

The retrospective approach may consist of having policies in place that require a scheduled review of accesses to records during a specified time period, a review in response to specific requests, or a review when misuse is suspected.

A prospective approach is more proactive and follows established algorithms designed to identify potential threats or breaches. Many organizations are now implementing newly available tools designed to provide proactive transaction log monitoring wherein alerts are issued for potential data access breaches in near real time.

Many of your policies relating to audit will be implemented via your technical security procedures. These will be based upon your privacy policies.

Questions to address as you develop Audit policies:
- What policies do you need to have in place to ensure that you can comply with a patient's request for an accounting of all accesses to his or her information?
- What policies do you need to ensure that you can identify (and respond) to real or potential privacy breaches?
- How will you assure that you can consistently locate and inspect which records have been accessed and by whom?

Accountability

Accountability refers to holding those responsible for security breaches—intentional or unintentional—liable for their actions. In the past, this was an often-overlooked area, and penalties were light or non-existent. Today, that is changing. The HITECH Act strengthens the penalties, which now include the possibility of fining organizations and individuals hundreds of thousands of dollars for intentional breaches with the intent to do harm. Even unintentional breaches are subject to fines. Various states have also added their own penalties for organizations and individuals. You need to pay close attention to these accountability requirements as you develop your own policies and procedures.

Your HIE policies not only need to cover the processes to protect a patient's information but also the actions you will take in response to various types of breaches.

Breaches can range from unintentional access, with no data actually viewed, to deliberate breaches with malicious intent.

Questions to address as you develop Accountability policies:

- How will you hold those responsible for security breaches liable for their actions in accordance with HIPAA and HITECH requirements?
- What are the various levels and types of breaches for which you will hold your participants accountable?
- What are your policies regarding patient notification of breaches?
- What are the penalties for privacy breaches? Are these penalties based upon whether the breach was intentional?
- Do the penalties take into account how much, if any, damage occurred?
- How, and when, are patients to be informed of privacy breaches of their personal health information?
- How will you hold those responsible for security breaches liable for their actions in accordance with HIPAA and HITECH requirements?

ACCEPTABLE USE OF PATIENT HEALTH INFORMATION (PHI)

The HITECH Act and other federal laws place strong emphasis on improving the quality of healthcare in the United States. One of the key initiatives to bring about this improvement is the ability to electronically collect health data so that the data can be de-identified, aggregated, and analyzed. This increased availability of data for analysis leads to questions around the appropriate use of health information.

You need specific policies that address how the data in your HIE will be used and what, if any, reuse of data will be allowed.

HIPAA specifically addresses the use and reuse of identifiable patient data. However, it is important to understand that there are many potential uses for de-identified data. Public health departments may request access to data for biosurveillance purposes intended for early detection of disease outbreaks. While providing data for public health purposes may be covered by state mandatory reporting laws, other requests may not be as clearly covered. Universities and other research organizations may request data for their own research purposes. Commercial entities may request data for research or marketing purposes. As you develop your data use and reuse policies you need to understand both relevant federal and state laws—*and* your stakeholders' desires.

It is critical that your policies on use and reuse of data comply not only with relevant laws but also reflect the sensitivities of your stakeholders. Your privacy policies must be transparent and must focus on maintaining the trust of your stakeholders.

Questions to address as you develop Acceptable Use policies:

- What are the applicable state and federal laws mandating sharing of the data, and how do your policies reflect compliance?
- What is your policy regarding providing federal, state, or local government access to data, and under what circumstances?
- What do your policies say about using HIE-stored data for research purposes? What types of research?
- Will you ever sell the de-identified data? And under what conditions?

- How do your privacy policies promote trust and transparency in regards to the use and reuse of the data in your HIE?

Business Associate Agreements and Covered Entities

Under HIPAA, HIEs are considered "Business Associates" of covered entities. HIPAA requires covered entities to contract with any entities to which they disclose Protected Health Information. The intent is to ensure that the data from a covered entity remain private and confidential.

The HITECH Act expands the HIPAA privacy and security regulations in three key areas related to business associates. Business associates now must (1) comply directly with Security Rule provisions directing implementation of administrative, physical, and technical safeguards for electronic protected health information; (2) comply with breach notification rules of the HITECH Act; and (3) HHS may now enforce a business associates' Security Rule obligation directly against the business associate. In addition, Business Associates are also covered under Privacy Rule sections focused on data use. In effect, these changes mean that HIEs must comply with the stricter regulations that were earlier put in place for covered entities.

Your success in getting a covered entity that will share information through your HIE to sign a Business Associate Agreement with the HIE starts early in your formation process. It begins with your earliest contacts with them and continues throughout your formation efforts. Figure 7-6 lists some of the steps to executing Business Associate Agreements.

To ensure participation, you must develop and proactively maintain positive and open relationships with, and the trust of, your stakeholders. We believe this means that you must involve your stakeholders in developing your policies, listen to their concerns

---

❑ 1. Research state and federal requirements for Business Associate Agreements.

❑ 2. Work with your state HIE collaborative (State Designated Entity) to understand your state's requirements regarding Business Associate Agreements. Many states are designing statewide agreements that can be used by all entities involved in sharing health information within the state.

❑ 3. Involve your key stakeholders as you create your policies and develop your approach to business associate agreements.

❑ 4. Discuss/negotiate agreements with the organizations you plan to involve in your HIE.

❑ 5. Obtain signed agreements.

Figure 7-6: Checklist—Developing and Executing Business Associate Agreements

- Multi-party agreement
- Identification of the participants
- Privacy and security obligations
- Requests for information based on permitted purposes
- Duty to respond
- Future use of data received through the NHIN
- Duties of requesting and responding participants
- Autonomy principle for access
- Responding participant's legal requirements
- Authorizations
- Participant breach notification
- Mandatory non-binding dispute resolution
- Allocation of liability risk

Figure 7-7: DURSA Components

and incorporate their feedback—long before you actually need to sign Business Associate Agreements with them or request that they share their information with your HIE.

The Data Use and Reciprocal Support Agreement (DURSA)

The DURSA[22] provides a good foundation for understanding the contractual rights of HIE participants. The DURSA was created by the NHIN demonstration projects for use by entities participating in the NHIN. It is a multi-party agreement that establishes the rules of engagement and obligations to which all NHIN participants must agree. All NHIN participants must sign the agreement as a condition of joining the community.

The DURSA is based upon an existing body of laws (federal, state, local) and the current policy framework. The agreement, while articulated as a contract, provides a framework for broad-based information exchange among a set of trusted entities. The agreement reflects a consensus of various federal, state, and private entities on the components listed in Figure 7-7.

PATIENT AND PROVIDER EDUCATION AND ENGAGEMENT

Privacy, as we said at the beginning of this chapter, is personal. There are constant reminders in the news media of the risk to patients from inappropriate disclosure of their personal information. Among the many things patients and consumers worry about, paramount are concerns as to how they can control access to their personal information and what would happen if their personal information got into the wrong hands. Their concerns are justified. For example, medical identify theft for fraudulent financial purposes is frequently in the news and is viewed by many as a growing problem.

Providers are concerned about the need to keep their patients' information confidential, especially if they share those data through an HIE. They need to understand how the HIE will maintain patient confidentiality when the data are shared. They need to understand what you are doing to protect patient privacy and how you will address any breaches of that privacy. Providers also have concerns about their potential liability for a privacy breach that occurs in an HIE environment. They may be skeptical about allowing the data they collect on patients to be used by others. They are also concerned about their personal and professional liability if the information they collected is subsequently misused—even if they are not in direct control of the data at the time of misuse.

It is crucial to involve your various stakeholders in discussions as you develop your organization's privacy policies. One of the best ways to ensure that people trust that their information will remain private is to proactively include them in the process of designing your privacy environment.

Solicit their input. Listen and respond to their concerns. Keep your stakeholders informed. Ensure that your policies and practices address their issues as completely as possible, and keep your privacy practices as transparent as possible.

Typically, stakeholders will need education to understand just what you will do with their data and how it will be handled. Your community may have specific consumer groups that are very sensitive about PHI or other nuances that will require specific dialogs around the subject of privacy. The best way to understand these concerns is to discuss them openly and directly. Communicate your interest in their concerns. Let them know that you are incorporating their input into the HIE policies and practices that you are developing. Provide consumer and provider education sessions.

As we've said before, trust is paramount to your success. Showing your stakeholders that you are interested in their concerns and that you are providing the necessary safeguards to ensure the privacy of their PHI is a top priority for you. They are necessary steps in your journey to a successful, sustainable HIE.

There are many resources available to assist you as you develop and implement your privacy education efforts. The federally sponsored HISPC initiative developed an excellent set of tools for consumer and provider education on privacy. These tools can be found on their website.[23] Other resources can be found at the end of this chapter.

The checklist in Figure 7-8 summarizes the steps you should include as you develop your approach to privacy.

RECAPPING THE "RIGHTS" OF PRIVACY

Ensuring the privacy of patient information can seem like a daunting endeavor. However, we have found that if you keep the following "rights" in mind, it will provide a good check to ensure you are doing the *"right" thing*. Your privacy policies need to ensure that your HIE data are accessed:

- By the *right* **person**
- With the *right* **access** privileges
- For the *right* **reasons**
- On the *right* **patient**
- With the *right* patient **consent**

❏ 1. Understand the landscape of privacy requirements.

❏ 2. Develop a broad understanding of HIPAA and other laws and regulations pertaining to the privacy of health information— including more stringent state laws.

❏ 3. Review privacy policies from other HIEs—particularly those with whom you are likely to exchange data.

❏ 4. Seek legal advice.

❏ 5. Involve your community of stakeholders to understand their privacy-related concerns and issues.

❏ 6. Inform and educate your stakeholders on the privacy work that you are doing.

❏ 7. Consult with your State Designated Entity.

❏ 8. Use stakeholder input to inform your policies.

❏ 9. Hold discussions among your workgroups and other stakeholders to determine the practicality and feasibility of your proposed policies.

❏ 10. Develop privacy policies that address the following key areas:
- Authentication
- Authorization
- Access to data
- Audit policies
- Accountability
- Data use and reuse

❏ 11. Work in collaboration with the security experts in the Technology & Security Workgroup to understand how technology can enable and support your privacy policies and ensure that those policies are both economically and technically feasible to implement.

❏ 12. Develop and document your policies and procedures.

❏ 13. Put the policies out for review by legal advisors, board members, and other stakeholders to provide an opportunity for discussion and modification.

❏ 14. Present your policies to your board for approval.

Figure 7-8: Checklist—Developing Good Privacy Policies

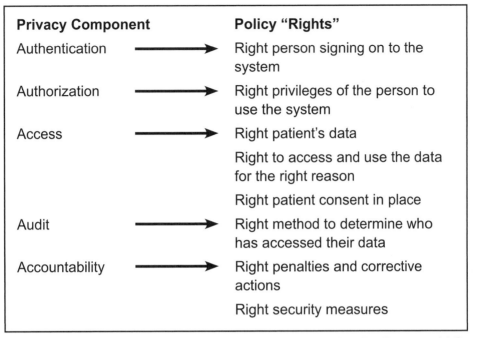

Privacy Component	Policy "Rights"
Authentication ⟶	Right person signing on to the system
Authorization ⟶	Right privileges of the person to use the system
Access ⟶	Right patient's data
	Right to access and use the data for the right reason
	Right patient consent in place
Audit ⟶	Right method to determine who has accessed their data
Accountability ⟶	Right penalties and corrective actions
	Right security measures

Figure 7-9: The 5 A's and the Policy "Rights." © 2010 Mosaica Partners, LLC. Used by permission.

Figure 7-9 summarizes these rights, as they are associated with the "5 A's."

Make certain that your privacy policies permeate throughout the rest of your HIE formation efforts. Your organization must be built on the principles of protecting patients' privacy. Remember, your providers and patients *will* take it personally.

WHOM TO INVOLVE

You need to seek legal advice from someone well acquainted with laws and regulations regarding the protection of health information and who is also well versed in the technology of HIEs. You will also need to involve representatives from your provider and consumer groups to assure that the policies being developed are acceptable to them and to the larger community.

It is also valuable to include someone with in-depth knowledge of security from a technical perspective. This person could be an individual certified in HIPAA or in privacy and security. While you will not want technical aspects alone to drive your policies, it is helpful to understand the technical implications of your privacy policies from both financial and implementation perspectives. You will also want to collaborate with the Technology & Security Workgroup to ensure there is alignment between the policies you develop and the technical security capabilities that are planned.

CHAPTER SUMMARY

In this chapter we have discussed how protecting patient privacy is critical to the success of an HIE. It is important, not only because federal and state laws require it, but because it is necessary to establish and maintain the trust of your stakeholders.

We provided a brief history of personal privacy protection of electronic information in the U.S. and addressed some of the relevant current federal regulations.

To assist you in understanding some of the areas to consider as you develop your privacy policies, we introduced the framework of the "5A's" of Security: Authentication, Authorization, Access, Audit, and Accountability. We also covered some of the issues relating to data use.

We discussed Business Associate Agreements and the associated responsibilities HIEs have, particularly in light of the modifications made to HIPAA by HITECH. Lastly, we provided a short discussion on the importance of educating your stakeholders on privacy. It is important that they are informed of your privacy policies and recognize that you understand and are addressing their concerns.

When you complete the activities addressed in this chapter you will have:

- A basic knowledge of the privacy environment in the U.S., especially as it relates to healthcare.
- An understanding of the framework upon which to create your HIE policies and procedures.
- Developed key privacy policies.
- Developed a plan to communicate and dialogue with your stakeholders on issues relating to the privacy of patient health information.

CASE STUDIES

HealthInfoNet

Devore Culver, Executive Director and CEO, HealthInfoNet

HealthInfoNet works closely with both the providers and their community at large on the issue of privacy. Their basic tenet is that neither patients nor providers release ownership of the data to the exchange. In this spirit, the contracts that they execute with their participants specifically define what the exchange can do with the data, and it is limited to use only for treatment. No data are released by the exchange unless it is confirmed that the requester is treating the patient.

In a "break-the-glass scenario," the provider goes through a process that establishes the provider's role and relationship to the patient and then validates that they have the patients' permission to access their data.

The state of Maine has modified its privacy laws to recognize Opt Out as the standard practice in the exchange of health information. This means that unless a person opts out of the exchange, their data are included.

HealthInfoNet implements this through providers who educate their patients and take on the responsibility of ensuring that patients are informed that their data will be sent to the exchange unless they specifically forbid it. The information about the exchange of data exists in all notices of privacy statements.

At HealthInfoNet, if a patient opts out of the exchange, any clinical content current in the exchange that is associated with the patient is purged. Subsequently, all clinical information associated with this patient is blocked from inclusion in the exchange. If, at a future point, a patient who has previously opted out of the exchange decides to include his or her information, only data from the date of change and forward are sent to the exchange. There is no retrospective loading of data.

CareSpark

Liesa Jenkins, Executive Director, CareSpark

Because CareSpark serves patients and providers in multiple states, they have adopted a model wherein each provider determines whether to implement an "opt-in" or "opt-out" approach. The HIE then honors the provider's approach.

According to an early survey of patients in which CareSpark asked them if they wanted their data shared, with whom it should be shared, and where they wanted to give permission for sharing their information:

- More than 90% of the respondents would grant access to their doctor, an emergency medical technician, and a family member.
- 50% would grant access to a public health agency.
- Only 20% would consent to sharing with employers and insurers.
- And 0% would grant consent for marketing purposes.

The survey also found that 90% of patients surveyed preferred to provide consent at the location at which they receive care.

At the time the provider sends the patient data, the provider logs on to CareSpark and indicates that the patient has consented to the sharing of information. This is then recorded both at the provider's office and with CareSpark's consent engine.

MedVirginia

Michael Matthews, CEO, MedVirginia

MedVirginia posts their privacy policies on their website. Briefly, these policies address:

- Requirement of a Business Associate Agreement for all participants;
- Access to data is limited to providers who have an established relationship with the patient;
- Additional security layers for information relating to HIV and psychotherapy;
- Verification of credential of healthcare providers;
- Limited access to physician practice notes; and
- Description of security safeguards in place.

MedVirginia was a participant in the NHIN Trial Implementation early on and continues to be active in NHIN-related initiatives. As part of their NHIN participation, a member of the MedVirginia team co-chaired the workgroup that created the Data Use and Reciprocal Support Agreement (DURSA). The DURSA includes a code of conduct that is required for participation in the NHIN.

The complete MedVirginia privacy policies are available online at http://www.medvirginia.net/privacy_security.html.

Rhode Island Quality Institute

Laura Adams, President and CEO, Rhode Island Quality Institute

As with many of the other successful HIEs, Laura Adams, CEO, Rhode Island Quality Institute, related how developing their privacy policies and practices involved a broad spectrum of stakeholders and legal counsel. Among those who participated in the development of privacy policies—and some of their concerns—were:

- American Civil Liberties Union (ACLU)—concern about putting sensitive information on the Internet, the control consumers would have over participating in the HIE and access to their information, and the regulatory framework that would govern the HIE.
- Rhode Island Coalition Against Domestic Violence—concern over protecting the rights of abused persons and sensitizing the community to the fact that, for an abused person, something as simple as disclosure of treatment of broken ribs could represent information that must be protected from exposure.
- Ethicists.
- Consumers and consumer advocacy groups.
- The Health Advocate in the Office of the Rhode Island Attorney General—concern in support of consumer protection.

The result of these meetings and dialogues was a consent model that must be voluntary for patients and providers. There are strong penalties for misuse—$10K per patient per incident of unauthorized access if convicted. Further, there is also immunity for providers that rely on the data coming out of the exchange, so they cannot be held liable if the data they receive are incorrect.

Consumers have considerable control over whether or not their information is included in the exchange. They must sign up to participate. Once consumers decide to participate in the exchange, all of their data are sent to the exchange. They do not have the ability to block individual information; however, they control who sees the data.

The enrollment process offers three consent options:

1. I authorize any and all health care providers/organizations who are treating me or are involved in the coordination of my health care to access any and all of my health information through **currrent*care***.

2. I authorize any and all health care providers/organizations access to my health information through **currrent*care*** only in an emergency or unscheduled event on a temporary basis.

3. I authorize the following health care providers/organizations to have access to my health information through **currrent*care***. (A list of specific providers/organizations would follow.)

Consumers may opt-in or opt-out at will, but if a consumer opts not to be in the exchange, there is no collection of their data during the time they were opted out, and no data will be gathered retrospectively.

The individual providers are collaborating to educate patients on the value of being in the exchange and obtaining their consent. Early focus groups of consumers indicated that the place where they felt most comfortable consenting to participation in an HIE was within the trusted relationship with their providers. Providers are paid $3 per enrolled consumer to reimburse them for the time spent educating patients about the exchange and their options for participation.

North Carolina Healthcare Information and Communications Alliance, Inc. (NCHICA)

Holt Anderson, Executive Director, North Carolina Healthcare Information and Communications Alliance

The North Carolina Healthcare Information and Communications Alliance, Inc. (NCHICA) was founded in 1994 by Executive Order of Governor James Hunt, Jr. For the past 16 years, NCHICA has promoted the use of information technology to improve healthcare, paving the way for the major ARRA HITECH initiatives today. While NCHICA itself is not an HIE, its workgroups and taskforces have developed many valuable tools that are available to organizations developing a health information exchange. Examples of resources related to privacy include:

- Model Business Associate Agreement (with supplemental materials)
- HITECH Act Breach Notification Risk Assessment Tool
- Notice of Privacy Practices

These and other HIPAA privacy and security resources are available online at http://www.nchica.org/HIPAAResources/security_privacy.htm.

State of Florida

Christopher Sullivan, PhD, Administrator, Agency for Health Care Administration

According to Christopher Sullivan, Florida has been very active in addressing and changing state laws that made it difficult to exchange electronic health information. Examples of some of that state's forward-thinking approach include:

- Up until 2008, Florida statute prohibited hospitals from sending patient records to providers other than those who were the admitting or attending providers during a specific episode of care, without patient consent. That has been changed to allow hospitals to send the data without consent.
- Another statute addressed allowed a laboratory to send results only to the ordering physician. Now labs can use an intermediary (such as an HIE) to send the results to the physician.

As an example of a leading practice, Florida has created a universal consent form, which is available online at http://168.82.75.17/PSresourceCtr/FLPSproject/ruledevelopment.shtml. A patient/provider can use this consent form to allow the release of a patient's information. If providers use this universal consent form, the law will provide to them immunity from consent liability.

RESOURCES

HIMSS. The HIMSS Privacy and Security Toolkit. http://www.himss.org/ASP/privacySecurityTree.asp?faid=78&tid=4#PSToolkitPSToolkit. Accessed April, 2010.

Markle Foundation. Connecting for Health Common Framework Policy Guides.
http://www.connectingforhealth.org/commonframework/index.html#guide. Accessed April, 2010.

Department of Health & Human Services. Business Associate Contracts. http://www.dhhs.gov/ocr/privacy/hipaa/understanding/coveredentities/contractprov.html. Accessed April, 2010.

Department of Health & Human Services, Privacy and Security (home page). http://healthit.hhs.gov/portal/server.pt?open=512&objID=1147&parentname=CommunityPage&parentid=0&mode=2&in_hi_userid=10741&cached=true. Accessed April, 2010.

Department of Health & Human Services, The Nationwide Privacy and Security Framework for Electronic Exchange of Individually Identifiable Health Information (home page). http://healthit.hhs.gov/portal/server.pt?open=512&mode=2&cached=true&objID=1173. Accessed April, 2010.

Department of Health & Human Services, HISPC Project State-Level Privacy and Security Resources. http://healthit.hhs.gov/portal/server.pt?open=512&objID=1175&parentname=CommunityPage&parentid=1&mode=2&in_hi_userid=10741&cached=true. Accessed April, 2010.

Department of Health & Human Services, The Nationwide Privacy and Security Framework for Electronic Exchange of Individually Identifiable Health Information. Posted December 15, 2009. http://healthit.hhs.gov/portal/server.pt/gateway/PTARGS_0_10731_848088_0_0_18/NationwidePS_Framework-5.pdf. Accessed April, 2010.

Department of Health & Human Services, Privacy Act of 1974. http://www.hhs.gov/foia/privacy/index.html. Accessed April, 2010.

Department of Health & Human Services, HIPAA Privacy Rule. http://www.hhs.gov/ocr/privacy/hipaa/administrative/privacyrule/adminsimpregtext.pdf. Accessed April, 2010.

Department of Health & Human Services, HHS Rule to impose stricter penalties for HIPAA violations to take effect November 30, 2009. http://edocket.access.gpo.gov/2009/E9-26203.htm. Accessed April, 2010.

Federal Information Security Management Act, 2002. http://aspe.hhs.gov/datacncl/Privacy/titleV.pdf. Accessed April, 2010.

Department of Health & Human Services, AHRQ HISPC Toolkit. http://healthit.ahrq.gov/portal/server.pt?open=514&objID=5562&mode=2&holderDisplayURL=http://prodportallb.ahrq.gov:7087/publishedcontent/publish/communities/a_e/ahrq_funded_projects/rti_toolkit/main/rti_toolkit.html. Accessed April, 2010.

Department of Health & Human Services, Understanding HIPAA Privacy Law – HHS. http://www.hhs.gov/ocr/privacy/hipaa/understanding/index.html. Accessed April, 2010.

REFERENCES

1. Department of Health, Education and Welfare. Report of the Secretary's Advisory Committee on Automated Personal Data Systems, Records, Computers, and the Rights of Citizens viii (1973). http://aspe.hhs.gov/DATACNCL/1973privacy/tocprefacememembers.htm. Accessed April, 2010.

2. Department of Health, Education and Welfare. The Code of Fair Information Practices. Posted 1973. http://www.epic.org/privacy/consumer/code_fair_info.html. Accessed April, 2010.

3. Markle Foundation. The Connecting for Health Common Framework: Resources for Implementing Private and Secure Health Information Exchange 2006.

4. Department of Justice website http://www.justice.gov/opcl/privacyact1974.htm. Accessed October, 2010.

5. Department of Health & Human Services. Health Information Privacy for Covered Entities. http://www.dhhs.gov/ocr/privacy/hipaa/understanding/coveredentities/index.html. Accessed April, 2010.

6. Department of Health & Human Services. HIPAA Administrative Simplification Regulation Text, 45 CFR Parts 160, 162, 164 (Unofficial Version as amended through February 16, 2006). http://www.hhs.gov/ocr/privacy/hipaa/administrative/index.html. Accessed April, 2010.

7. 45CFR.164.506.

8. Department of Health & Human Services. Summary of Selected Federal Laws and Regulations Addressing Confidentiality, Privacy and Security. http://healthit.hhs.gov/portal/server.pt/gateway/PTARGS_0_11113_911059_0_0_18/Federal%20Privacy%20Laws%20Table%202%2026%2010%20Final.pdf. Accessed April, 2010.

9. Department of Health & Human Services. Privacy and Security Home Page. http://healthit.hhs.gov/portal/server.pt?open=512&objID=1147&parentname=CommunityPage&parentid=0&mode=2&in_hi_userid=10741&cached=true. Accessed April, 2010.

10. Federal Trade Commission Act, http://www.ftc.gov/ogc/ftcact.shtm. Accessed April, 2010.

11. Senate Banking Committee, http://banking.senate.gov/conf/confrpt.htm. Accessed October, 2010.

12. Sarbanes Act of 2002. http://uscode.house.gov/download/pls/15C98.txt. Accessed October, 2010.

13. PCI Security Standards Council. https://www.pcisecuritystandards.org/index.shtml. Accessed October, 2010.

14. Department of Education. http://www2.ed.gov/policy/gen/guid/fpco/ferpa/index.html. Accessed October, 2010.

15. Department of Labor. http://www.dol.gov/ebsa/compliance_assistance.html. Accessed October, 2010.

16. Department of Heath & Human Services. Privacy and Security Framework. http://healthit.hhs.gov/portal/server.pt?open=512&objID=1173&parentname=CommunityPage&parentid=3&mode=2&in_hi_userid=10741&cached=true. Accessed April, 2010.

17. HIMSS. Privacy and Security Toolkit. http://www.himss.org/ASP/privacySecurityTree.asp?faid=78&tid=4. Accessed April, 2010.

18. Department of Health & Human Services. Health Information Privacy, Health Information Technology. http://www.hhs.gov/ocr/privacy/hipaa/understanding/special/healthit/index.html. Accessed April, 2010.

19. HIMSS. *HIMSS Dictionary of Healthcare Information Technology Terms, Acronyms and Organizations.* Chicago: HIMSS; 2010.

20. Interview with Devore Culver, Executive Director and CEO, HealthInfoNet, April, 2010.

21. HITECH, Section 13405(c).

22. NHIN Cooperative DURSA Workgroup. Data Use and Reciprocal Support Agreement (DURSA). Posted January 23. http://healthit.hhs.gov/portal/server.pt/gateway/PTARGS_0_11673_909240_0_0_18/DURSAVersionforProductionPilotsFinal.pdf. Accessed April, 2010.

23. Department of Health & Human Services. The Health Information Privacy and Security Collaboration (HISPC). http://healthit.hhs.gov/portal/server.pt?open=512&mode=2&cached=true&objID=1240. Accessed April, 2010.

CHAPTER 8

The Time for Technology

*Your HIE needs to be driven by your community's values,
not by a technology vendors' solutions and staff.*

INTRODUCTION

This chapter on technology is intentionally placed near the end of the book. Before you make any decisions concerning specific technology, you should have an organization in place, a business model created, sources of funding identified—and ideally committed—and most important of all, you must know what services your stakeholders have indicated they want you to provide.

While it is true that you need to begin early in the formation process with educating yourself on HIE technology strategies and technical approaches—as well as various vendor products for exchanging health information—to inform your budget planning, do not be seduced into treating your HIE formation as a technology project. *It is not.*

Forming an HIE is a major change management project—one whose successful completion is enabled by technology. Revisit your vision and mission often to keep focused:

> **Caution**
>
> Do not allow an early request for technology cost estimates to drive you prematurely into a technical discussion or decision.

Your HIE's champions—those stakeholders who have been open and vocal about supporting you—can be of great assistance as you navigate through your choices and discussions regarding technology by helping to limit scope creep and by keeping the process focused on what is important: providing value for all of your stakeholders, including the patients.

The purpose of technology in your HIE is to automate the capabilities that must be in place to securely and accurately share patient health information and support the services you offer. In this chapter, we discuss the technical components and processes that you need to have in place to implement cross-organizational data sharing. The good news is that while complex, the choice and implementation of technology is a mature area, and there are a lot of resources available to help you.

This chapter begins with a brief discussion of the business services and capabilities that are supported by many of today's HIEs. Regardless of the services and capabilities that you decide to provide through your HIE, your technology strategy and solutions must support these business services. Also, you need to identify early on the associated technical implications and potential challenges that you will face as you move forward. We go on to discuss the attributes or the characteristics that must define your technical environment to ensure that patient privacy is maintained through your implementation of appropriate security controls. Finally, we discuss some of the methods for choosing and acquiring HIE services, the technologies that support those services, and the questions you need to consider in developing your technology approach and in making technology decisions.

SECURITY

> **Caution**
>
> A system which provides impenetrable, perfect, automated security is neither financially nor practically feasible for your organization.

Generally, you will hear privacy and security referred to together, as though they were one and the same. As mentioned in Chapter 7, *Protecting Patient Privacy*, we have intentionally separated security from the discussion of privacy. Ensuring privacy—of personal health information (PHI)—is the goal. It is what you need to assure your stakeholders you are protecting. Security, on the other hand, consists of the processes and technology capabilities you put in place to achieve your goal of ensuring privacy.

The **objective of security** in the healthcare environment is to ensure that personally identifiable health information is protected with reasonable administrative, technical, and physical safeguards to ensure its confidentiality, integrity, and availability and to prevent its unauthorized or inappropriate access, use, modification, or disclosure. Your security policies and procedures describe how your information and systems are protected from unauthorized access, use, disclosure, disruption, modification, or destruction. They include how the data are protected, both while it is at rest or stored, as well as during transmission.

Use your privacy policies, developed in conjunction with your stakeholders, to inform your security requirements. Then further refine the requirements in your security policies and procedures. These will drive your security-related technology investments. Your security practices are the tangible implementation of many of your privacy policies.

A word of caution: Impenetrable, perfect, automated security is neither financially viable nor practically feasible for your organization. You will have to make decisions regarding the trade-offs between automation, manual procedures, and cost. At a minimum, you should automate some, if not all, of the authentication, authorization, and access control processes. These areas should be addressed in the security risk assessment, which can also include additional recommendations for the HIE, such as including an automated proactive auditing and alerting process.

Developing and implementing technical security controls requires that you engage an expert in health IT security, as well as someone well versed in privacy law. Expect to have lively discussions as you develop your security policies and procedures and select

---

Authentication

Ensuring that individuals logging into the system are who they say they are.

Authorization

Determining that individuals are allowed to access the HIE.

Access to Data

Determining to which data the person has access and what actions they are allowed to take relative to that data.

Audit

Ensuring that you can consistently inspect what records have been accessed and by whom.

Accountability

Determining how you will hold those responsible for security breaches liable.

Figure 8-1: The 5 A's of Security

the technical tools required for implementation. This can be a time of fantastic learning and growth for your organization.

The 5 A's

Previously, we discussed the "5 A's" in terms of their relationship to developing privacy policies. Here we discuss them in terms of their security implications related to specific services and capabilities that the technology must support. These are the attributes around which you need to develop specific policies and procedures to protect the patient's right to privacy of their PHI. The job of the Technology & Security Workgroup is to define and implement the technology infrastructure that both enables the business services and protects an individual's privacy.

Technical security is a broad and deep field. In this chapter, we provide a basic framework that describes the various issues you need to address. The resource list at the end of the chapter will point you to sources for additional, more in-depth, technical information. As a reminder, the "5 A's of Security," first discussed in Chapter 7, *Protecting Patient Privacy*, are shown again in Figure 8-1.

ESSENTIAL HIE SERVICES AND CAPABILITIES

Every HIE must have a basic set of capabilities in place before they can become operational and provide services. Some of these capabilities are technology-based. How you develop or acquire these capabilities is determined by your policies, budget, stakeholder wants and needs, and the services offered. Only when you fully understand the broad range of capabilities and services that you need to support your stakeholders—and the constraints within which the services will be provided—are you ready to acquire and

---

Examples of HIE Security-Related Services

1. Correctly identify and authenticate a user of the system.

2. Ensure that data are accessed appropriately and used only for the right reasons (authorization and consent).

3. Correctly identify a patient.

4. Correctly locate the relevant data sources.

5. Accurately retrieve data from multiple sources.

6. Accurately send data to multiple sources.

7. Aggregate patient data.

8. Ensure that data provided to the requestor are an accurate representation of the data received from the data source(s).

9. Provide patients with a complete list of successful exchanges of their data upon request.

10. Ensure that the organization is able to identify and hold accountable those who misuse data.

Other HIE Services

1. Appropriately present patient data in a meaningful way.

2. Provide a central access point for data requests.

3. Provide the services and support that are required for the business within agreed upon time frames.

Figure 8-2: Typical HIE Services

implement technology. Figure 8-2 lists some typical services and capabilities found in successful HIEs.

All of these services must be present in an environment that, first and foremost, protects the patient's privacy.

ESSENTIAL SERVICES AND THE SECURITY AND TECHNICAL IMPLICATIONS

The following section describes how the services you provide and the security and technology you implement must be woven together to provide a robust, secure technical platform for HIE. In this section we address in more detail the following services:

- Correctly identify and authenticate a user of the system.
- Ensure that data are accessed appropriately and used only for the right reasons.
- Correctly identify the patient.
- Correctly locate relevant data sources.
- Retrieve data from multiple sources.
- Send data to multiple sources.

- Meaningful aggregation of patient data.
- Provide patients with a complete list of successful (and approved) exchanges of their data upon request.
- Auditing capabilities that enable organizations to hold accountable those who misuse data.

Correctly Identify and Authenticate a User of the System

Ensuring that individuals requesting access to the HIE are who they claim to be is a critical component of your security.

Authentication

Authentication is a method of validating that users are who they claim to be. Authentication is made up of two processes: it begins with how users are first identified within their own technical domain before they are given HIE access privileges. Identification can be as simple as allowing the user to claim an identity, or as complicated as requiring a complete security background check. Identification typically is driven by the security levels of the data users will be accessing. Healthcare typically requires a form of state-issued identification to verify a person's identity, and for physicians, typically adds the requirement for verification of a medical license. However, as an individual's identity is established, it is important that a record is kept of the specific identity verification process used, and the identifying and background data gathered, in case of any breach subsequently attributed to the individual.

Once an individual's identity is verified, the typical process involves assigning a unique personal identifier* and a password known only to the individual. In practice, the personal identifier will often be an employee ID number, or, possibly, a login name guaranteed unique within the scope of the authenticating technical domain. Typically, the password will be issued as a system-generated one-time password, which is required to be changed on the first login event, thereby guaranteeing that the password is not known to anyone (including the issuing authority) other than the owner of the identifier.

The second process related to Authentication is the actual use of the identifier and password when a user desires access to the computer system. The user typically enters his or her identifier and is then challenged with a request for a password which, when entered, is obscured from view to protect against it being viewed by someone in close proximity to the login screen. In this manner, the user can be verified since the identifier is unique, and the password is known only to that individual.

Other factors can also be used as a replacement for, or in addition to, the secret password. There are three types of authentication "factors" that can be used during the authentication process. These can be used either individually, or in combination: (1) something the person knows such as a secret password or key phrase; (2) something the person possess such as a token, key card, or radio-frequency identification (RFID) tag; and (3) something physical about the person such as a fingerprint, voiceprint, or reti-

---

* An identifier is an attribute that points unambiguously and uniquely to a specific person or entity.

nal image. A common way to make the authentication process stronger is to require two different factors be employed before allowing access (called 2-factor authentication).

> **For example:** To withdraw cash from an ATM, individuals insert their ATM bank-card (something they have) and enter their PIN (something they know). This is a form of 2-factor authentication.

Properly implemented, authentication policies, along with the appropriate technology solutions, will provide a high level of protection against fraudulent use. You need to determine the type and relative strength of authentication you will use to identify and authenticate users who will be accessing the HIE from a variety of entities around your community or state. The new regulations from the FDA for e-prescribing of controlled substances require a minimum of 2-factor authentication.

Ensure Data Are Accessed Appropriately and Used Only for the Right Reasons

There are two facets to the authorization to access data. The user must have the appropriate authorization to access the data, and the appropriate patient consent must have been obtained.

Authorization

Authorization is the process of determining what activities an authenticated user is permitted to perform or what services the user is allowed to access. The responsibility of the HIE is to understand and implement the appropriate access control tools and procedures to ensure that only appropriate access to information is granted when requests originate from a variety of access points. You need to determine that the person is allowed access to data through the HIE and exactly what types of data they are allowed to access.

Access to Data

Access to data is granted based upon the user's authorization to access the data and the level of consent that is in place from the patient. Once the system has validated that the person is who he or she claims to be and that he or she is authorized to request data, the system then must determine specifically which data that person is allowed to access. Access rights specifically define what data a person is allowed to access and what operations they may perform on the accessed data. Allowed actions may include view only, create, modify, delete, or some combination thereof.

Access is commonly implemented through a technical access control service (ACS) which includes embedded security management capabilities along with other access control and decision-making capabilities. The ACS is responsible for creating trust credentials that are used by the various organizational systems participating in the HIE to ensure that the proper level of authorization has been validated for any user accessing data in the system.

Many organizations use a process known as "role-based" access control that associates the person's identifier with various levels of access and permitted activities—roles. With this approach, each person (identifier) is assigned one or multiple roles. Each role has specifically defined rights of access to and actions upon data in the system.

Generally, role-based access is granted through multiple layers of specificity. A person is assigned a role(s), which is related to their need to access data types, and that role has access rights relating to what actions may be performed on which data. Then, depending on additional criteria, the roles become more granular and specific to the types of data that may be accessed and the allowed actions on the data.

> **For example:** A care provider could be assigned the role of "physician" or "radiology technician," depending on what is appropriate. The physician role will most likely have the right to full access of a patient's clinical information, but the level and types of data accessed depend upon many criteria, including the type of physician, the care setting, and the relationship of the physician to a particular patient. The radiology technician, on the other hand, may have access only to small portions of the patient's record that are necessary for the technician to complete and document the specific procedures for which he/she is responsible.

Correctly Identify the Patient

The goal of patient identification is the accurate identification of the patient and the correct linking of all related information to that individual within and across systems.

Patient Identity Integrity

A basic requirement for any successful HIE is the ability to correctly identify the patient for whom information is being requested. Correctly identifying each patient within your HIE requires that you provide Patient Identity (PI) Integrity or a Patient Identity Matching service. Your HIE must have that capability. Here we highlight some of the basic requirements for patient identity matching and discuss some of the current barriers to absolute certainty regarding a patient's identity when dealing with information that comes from multiple sources. For more in-depth information on the topic, we refer you to an excellent white paper, "Patient Identity Integrity,"[1] produced by the HIMSS Patient Identity Workgroup.

PI Integrity refers to the accuracy and completeness of data that is attached to, or associated with, an individual patient. Data must be reliable, reproducible, and sufficiently extensive for matching purposes. Completeness of data not only refers to having adequate data elements present but also to the correct linking of all existing records for an individual—within and across various information systems. PI Integrity is critical to ensuring accuracy and completeness of patient information.

Many of the activities of an HIE involve the exchange of clinical information between independent entities that typically use different methods for patient identification. The ability to correctly identify a patient in your HIE environment is a critical capability that your HIE must implement. The inability to ensure the accurate identification of a patient will result in a lack of trust in your HIE by your stakeholders.

Without PI Integrity in an HIE, information pertaining to an individual may exist in one or multiple databases (where it resides as a duplicate), be inaccessible, or remain unknown to those needing to see the complete or most current picture of a patient. Or, conversely, in the absence of PI Integrity, information on two individuals may be combined erroneously into one record.

Unique Individual Identifier

Some believe that in a perfect world we would have a unique identifier for each person. A unique identifier has the following characteristics: (1) it is linked to only one individual; (2) it provides unambiguous identification; (3) it is immutable over time with consistent syntax; (4) it is simple to implement; and (5) it is cost-effective when compared with other solutions. The advantages of a unique identifier for each individual have been appreciated by many for a long time. In 1996, HIPAA mandated a Unique Individual Identifier for healthcare purposes; however, there is a current Congressional proscription against using national unique identifiers in the U.S.[2] Due to public concerns over privacy, Congress prohibited HHS from using its authority under HIPAA to issue a final rule or standard. Progress on defining and establishing a unique identifier solution has been slow to almost non-existent due to concerns about the cost to implement, potential privacy risks in amassing large centralized databases, and technical issues on compatibility with existing systems, as well as a lack of national consensus on what identifier to use.

Unfortunately, we do not live in a perfect world. In reality, a unique identifier can only work when the identifier is immutable and always reproducible, and that has so far been difficult, if not impossible, to achieve. Therefore, we must strive to achieve the accuracy of a unique identifier with the tools and methods we currently have available. While in the U.S. we cannot have a national unique identifier, there is no prohibition against state- or regional-level unique identifiers.

Maintaining the integrity of your HIE's unique identifiers requires that you create the appropriate business processes. This includes identifying the workflow, policies, and procedures to ensure PI Integrity. This becomes challenging when considered in the context of an HIE record. Your governance and stewardship discussions, as well as policy development and execution, must involve a multi-stakeholder group that has executive-level involvement and support. Authority must be assigned within each organization that is participating in your HIE for ensuring active and ongoing oversight of patient identity management.

While maintaining PI Integrity is complex, there are many vendors that offer tools that can help you address patient identify management. For example, the Patient Identity and Administration profiles created by the Integrating the Healthcare Enterprise[3] (IHE) Initiative address transactions that relate to patient registration, coordination, and discharge. The NHIN has adopted some of these profiles to facilitate information exchange between HIE organizations that participate in the trial implementations.

IHE integration profiles serve as a foundation for leveraging and aggregating patient information. The profiles are technology agnostic and can be implemented in most vendor applications, but it requires the cooperation of the vendor, and their compliance needs to be assured through rigorous testing and contracting. HIMSS hosts an annual "Connect-a-Thon"[4] during which multiple vendors can participate and demonstrate that their products follow the current specifications.

Standardizing patient identification attributes and valuations increases the usability of the IHE profiles, simplifies queries between applications, and enables better identity matching processes. However, additional standards are required to support priorities within the broader healthcare and public health community.

Master Patient Index

The tool commonly used to implement patient identity matching is referred to as the Master Patient Index (MPI). Also referred to as the Master Person Index, this critical tool provides the capability to uniquely identify a patient across multiple information systems.

Most MPIs work by matching a set of information, known to be related to a specific person, to data contained in another record. The minimum data set for patient identification most commonly used in the industry includes full legal name (first, middle, last, suffix), date of birth (DOB), gender, full mailing address, and home telephone number. Generally, the MPI service is provided at a central location in the HIE. In some cases, states are developing a single statewide MPI, while others leave it to the regions. Check with your State Designated Entity to find out what your state is doing in this regard. You may be able to use the services of your state's statewide MPI.

Methods Used for Patient Matching

There are various technical methods, based on algorithmic formulas, that are used to match and link patient data. The three critical areas that impact the quality of this process are: (1) the quality of the data used for matching; (2) the quality of implementation of the matching criteria; and (3) the effectiveness of the actual algorithm itself.

Statistical or mathematically-based algorithms are dependent upon key demographic data points, as mentioned earlier, for a person or patient. These demographic attributes, such as name, DOB, and address are not unique to a single individual and, with the exception of DOB, frequently may change throughout a person's lifetime. This means that matching errors will continue to occur even when the matching algorithm is robust and standardized. Most matching algorithms perform better when they have more data elements available for comparison. Additional data, such as race or ethnicity, guarantor, insurance, next of kin, emergency contact, other identifiers (insurance number, driver's license number), mother's name, father's name, and work address, may also be collected. All of these data elements can be used by sophisticated statistical matching algorithms to improve the accuracy of patient record matching.

Although extremely accurate, no MPI matching algorithm is 100% accurate. A tool that uses a probabilistic algorithm for matching will allow you to set a predefined level of certainty that you will accept to determine that a particular record belongs to a specific patient. Any record whose probability falls below the preset limit for certainty, but is above a limit for likelihood, can then be presented for human review and decision.

Correctly Locate Relevant Data Sources

Record Locator Service (RLS)

Once a patient is identified, his or her medical records must be located. The record locator service (RLS) complements and operates in conjunction with the MPI service to direct requests for patient data to the [participating] locations holding those data.[5] The RLS serves as a registry of clinical activity about a patient that can include an entry for each visit—typically listing the providers, services delivered, and identifiers used in the source systems. It is used to identify all the participating locations that house information relating to a patient.

As you can see, the MPI and the RLS are tightly coupled. As with the MPI, the RLS is generally housed in a central location. When a request for information is received by the HIE, the MPI engine determines the identity of the person for whom information is being requested, and the RLS identifies where the various sources of information on that patient reside.

Retrieve Data from Multiple Sources and Send Data to Multiple Sources

A primary purpose of your HIE is to search for, and retrieve patient data from, multiple data suppliers and send it to the data requester. From a technical standpoint, there are three basic Health Information Exchange models to accomplish this: (1) the Centralized model; (2) the De-centralized or Federated model; and (3) the Hybrid model. The model that you choose for your HIE is dependent upon several factors, but most importantly, it is dependent upon the needs and desires of the stakeholders you serve and their willingness to share information.

Communities and providers typically differ in their policies and tolerance for maintaining direct control over the data they generate on a patient. Many providers are willing to send their data to a shared repository from which requests are handled for the providers from a central location (Centralized model). Other providers want to maintain direct control over the data at all times and only respond to direct requests (De-centralized or Federated model). Many communities find that the preferences of the providers vary from organization to organization and so the right model for them is a combination of the Centralized and De-Centralized model – known as the Hybrid model.

The architecture model you choose will most likely combine elements of more than one of these models. As with most things, there are variations within each of these models, but by far the most common models we see for HIEs today are the Centralized and Hybrid models.

Centralized Exchange Model

The Centralized Architecture model, shown in Figure 8-3, stores all the data determined to be eligible for exchange, from all providers participating in the exchange, in a central repository. Data from separate source organizations are not necessarily comingled, but there is a central repository to which the data are sent and from which the requested data are retrieved.

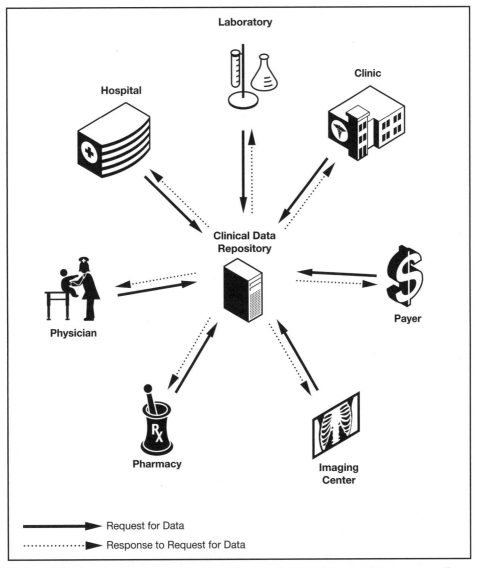

Figure 8-3: Centralized Architecture Model. © 2009 Mosaica Partners, LLC. Used by permission.

In the Centralized model, organizations proactively send their data to the central repository regardless of whether particular data have been requested by another organization. There is up-front agreement by the participating organizations and their patients on which data will be shared and under what circumstances. The original data continues to reside at the source organization, while the HIE retains a copy which it uses to respond to requests.

One advantage of this type of model is the speed at which the HIE can respond to data requests. Obviously, if the data are already located in one central repository, there is no lag time associated with the RLS searching various external locations for the appropriate records and data. Having the data in a central repository is also conducive to the aggregation of de-identified data for the purposes of research or reporting and the process for correcting or updating data is somewhat straight-forward. Data are generally available 24 hours a day, 7 days a week, as long as the central repository itself remains online.

One of the concerns often voiced relating to the Centralized model is that this architecture is at higher risk for security attacks and breaches, since it contains all of the data from many sources. Therefore, the value of such a target is much greater than the value of the individual data suppliers.

Another potential concern is that since the data are housed in one location, the consequences of a single point of failure are more far-reaching. Extra attention must be given to mitigating these risks. A key drawback to the Centralized model is the cost of implementation and support, which includes capital outlay for equipment, physical facilities, and resources.

De-centralized or Federated Model

The De-centralized Architecture model, also known as the Federated model, is, in essence, the opposite of the Centralized model (see Figure 8-4). In the De-centralized model, there is no central storage of data. In fact, in the extreme versions of this model, each request is sent to *every* potential source of data. If a data source has records for the requested individual, these records are sent directly to the requesting entity where they are typically processed for presentation to the requestor. In this approach, the HIE's role may be only to process the information request (broadcast the request to participants) and activate the search and retrieval of data. This logical model for exchange is actually the architecture used by the NHIN for locating and retrieving data from various HIEs.

Some De-centralized models may keep a central record of the locations of data they have accessed in previous inquiries, but this record consists only of the patient identifier and pointers to the data. No clinical data are stored centrally, but even having this level of information stored centrally makes this model a form of Hybrid model rather than a fully de-centralized one.

In Federated models, each organization implements an "edge" server that is located in a special firewall system. Typically, the edge server is located in what is referred to as the "DMZ" or an area between firewalls. One firewall is between the edge server and the outside world while the other firewall is between the edge server and the organization's internal system. This edge server processes the incoming requests for data, retrieves the data from the organization's internal systems or data that has been copied into the edge server's technical domain, packages it, and sends it directly to the requesting technical domain or organization, which in turn sends it to the internal requester.

A key characteristic of the De-centralized Architecture model is that the patient's data always remain with the source, and copies are sent to individual requesters only in direct response to queries. The receiving organization may store the data or present it for one-time viewing and then discard it.

An HIE can use a "push" model (source sends data to receiver without first receiving a request) for messaging or a "pull" model (data sent in response to a request). The push model may be an option to handle most, if not all of the Phase 1 Meaningful Use*

* See Chapter 1 for more information on the Meaningful Use Incentive Program.

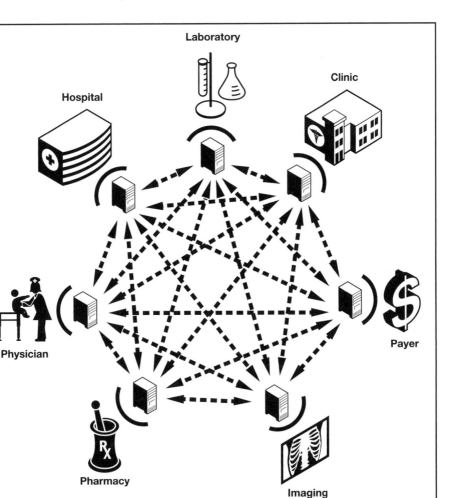

Laboratory

Clinic

Hospital

Physician

Payer

Pharmacy

Imaging
Center

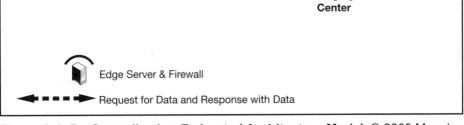

Edge Server & Firewall

Request for Data and Response with Data

Figure 8-4: De-Centralized or Federated Architecture Model. © 2009 Mosaica Partners, LLC. Used by permission.

requirements. For the push model, the Federated Architecture works well. The data sender knows the address, or queries the HIE for the address of the recipient, and the parties have reciprocal sharing agreements in place. Each participant provides a port to receive and process the data. In the simplest form of the Federated model, the messages are sent directly between participants.

One key advantage to the Federated model is that each organization maintains total control over their data. Another perceived advantage is that since there is no central storage of clinical data, the risk of a security breach that accesses aggregated clinical data from across the community is significantly reduced, or non-existent.

A significant disadvantage is associated with the sheer number of requests each organization needs to process. In addition, the question of how to replicate the data environment that was used to make clinical decisions must be addressed. This places the burden of preserving the "display instance" (information displayed at a particular point in time) on the requesting organization.

Another potential drawback of this model is the lag time between requests for data and the receipt of the complete data set. This lag may result in piecemeal data arriving at the requester at different times, which can affect the reliability and completeness of data. The availability of timely data relies on the operating practices and agreements with each participating data supplier and is subject to planned and unplanned outages at those entities.

Correcting and updating data poses additional questions, such as how an update can be replicated across all parties that previously received a copy of the original data. The recipient must also develop a process for responding to changes in data if they "persist," or retain, the data for future use. These are vital questions that must be addressed, as trust in the reliability, accuracy, and completeness of data is a vital component for physician participation and, ultimately, the success of the HIE.

Hybrid Model

In the Hybrid model, shown in Figure 8-5, there is a centralized MPI and RLS for identifying patients and locating data sources. As with the Centralized model, some organizations may proactively send their clinical data to a central repository, while others, as in the Federated model, are queried on an as-needed basis.

The Hybrid Architecture model, as you might expect, contains some characteristics of the Centralized model and some characteristics of the Federated model. For example, in this model, some data may be stored centrally, such as laboratory data that are regularly "pushed" to the HIE, while other data, such as pharmacy data, may be stored at the source and be available by request. Most Hybrid model HIEs will include some form of MPI services and an RLS, and many also perform centralized user authentication and authorization. Hybrid models also maintain a log of the data sources found as a result of information requests, and those that also handle clinical data will generally include information relative to the types of data exchanged.

One of the advantages of the Hybrid model is that it is flexible enough to meet a wide range of preferences of the participants relating to their choice of how they want to exchange data. Challenges arise in managing the various types of connections and updates or changes to data.

MedVirginia implemented a Centralized model for its regional exchange. They are operational with a current database holding information on 938,000 unique patients. MedVirginia was the first HIE in production on the NHIN, in partnership with the Social Security Administration (SSA), to automate the disability determination process. To share information with the SSA, they must accommodate the NHIN federated approach. As such, they function as a node on the national network. This is one example of a truly federated approach to sharing information.

MedVirginia is the sole private sector participant in the Hampton Roads VLER Community project. VLER, or Virtual Lifetime Electronic Records, is an initiative of

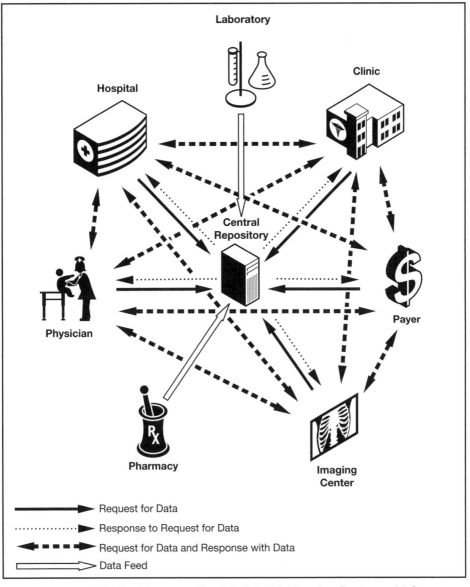

Figure 8-5: Hybrid Architecture Model. © 2009 Mosaica Partners, LLC. Used by permission.

both the Departments of Veterans Affairs and Defense to establish interoperability between their health records systems and with private sector healthcare providers.

Through funding from the Commonwealth of Virginia, MedVirginia provides health IT support to safety net providers in central Virginia. Capabilities include scheduling, results reporting, clinical documentation, and secure clinical messaging.

While understanding these various models and their implications may seem overwhelming if you are not a technology professional, rest assured that as you hold discussions with credible, experienced technology vendors and experts, you will be assured by their ability to fully explain how their product works and answer all of your questions. It is important for your HIE to have the technical strategy and approach identified (one that supports your service offerings) before beginning discussions with vendors. We have presented this brief overview to help you begin to understand the types of questions you need to consider as you move forward.

Meaningful Aggregation of Patient Data

Interoperability

Your stakeholders' trust in the accuracy of the data is paramount to your success. In healthcare, this requires that the data not only be accurate, but also that the meaning of the data be clear and unambiguous. To reliably share health information electronically, there must be a way to ensure that the data format and the meaning of the data are recorded and communicated accurately between multiple systems using different products. This is referred to as *semantic interoperability*.

> **For example:** Transmitting data associated with laboratory test results is necessary, but it is not sufficient for full meaning. For lab data to have meaning, the "normal ranges" for the data that are used by the testing lab must also accompany the data. For the data to be useful, it must retain its original meaning from the time when it was first captured.

The way the industry is approaching the solution to this problem is through setting standards and certification criteria for technical interoperability. Later in this chapter, we provide a summary of many of the key organizations that are involved in setting these standards and some of those responsible for certifying compliance with the established standards.

Standards

No chapter on technology would be complete without mentioning the many issues relating to standards. As the well-known saying goes, "There is no problem finding standards [in HIT]—there are lots to choose from."

> The lack of common consistent technical standards is a key barrier preventing the seamless electronic flow of health information today.

It is beyond the scope of this chapter, and indeed this book, to completely detail all of the relevant technical standards—and the specifics of those standards—for HIE. What we do provide, however, is a discussion to acquaint you with the key concepts of standards, an explanation of why you must pay close attention to their development and use, and the role they play in your technology procurement and implementation. We also provide a list of resources that supply you with in-depth information on this topic.

In the not-too-distant past, most health IT application developers—whether vendors or in-house IT departments—for the most part independently defined how their data were stored and transmitted. Even those who used external standards frequently modified them in their implementation. This prevalence of proprietary and "one-off" standards is one of the most significant technical barriers to HIE.

Thanks to the efforts of thousands of people across many different initiatives, a good deal of progress has been made in establishing standards in recent years. As discussed in Chapter 1, *The HIE Landscape*, at the federal level, HITSP was leading the effort. Other key organizations, including the Object Management Group (OMG), Health Level 7 (HL7), the American National Standards Institute (ANSI), and many others who have also made significant contributions. Things are getting better.

Figure 8-6 provides a summary of some of the key organizations involved in defining and setting standards, making them useful, and certifying their proper use. All of these efforts are aimed at one goal: improving the acceptance and use of common standards to more effectively share health information and improve care.

As you investigate and select the technology approach and technology vendor(s) to support your HIE, it is important that you are aware of the state of standards setting and adoption. Table 8-1 lists some of the more common data and messaging standards in use in health IT today.

Liesa Jenkins, Executive Director, CareSpark, is a firm believer in building the HIE on standards. CareSpark is unique among the early HIEs in that they built their technical infrastructure from the beginning on the IHE framework. According to Jenkins, this has enabled them to be more easily interoperable with the NHIN. When considering vendors for their HIE, they considered only those who used the IHE profiles, demonstrated interoperability, and were committed to a standards-based platform.

Many of the members of your Technology & Security workgroup will have in-depth experience and expertise in the health IT standards environment. They will provide much insight and knowledge that will guide you through your technology selection process. We also provide additional references at the end of this chapter.

Provide Patients with a Complete List of Successful (and Approved) Exchanges of Their Data upon Request

Audit

As mentioned previously in this book, HITECH requires that patients must be allowed to know who has accessed their personal health information and for what purposes. At the time of writing, this part of the law has not been finalized in regulations, so it is not yet known exactly how broadly and deeply the term "access" will be interpreted.

Creating an audit trail is a common method for tracking access to information. An audit trail enables the reconstruction of all activity within a system. For those organizations that currently use automated EHRs, this information has typically been accessed through the individual system audit logs. This provides a retrospective view of accesses but does not provide a mechanism for preventing inappropriate access. However, there are new tools on the market that use sophisticated algorithms for monitoring of logs and system activity in near real time to alert security officers of potential data breach situations.

HITECH strengthened security regulations and penalties under HIPAA. Organizations and individuals are now facing stiffer penalties for security breaches. It is a leading practice to automate as much of the review of your system logs as possible.

Well-prepared audit processes typically provide for the independent review and examination of records to make sure that the policies and procedures established by

Examples of Standards Setting Organizations

ANSI – American National Standards Institute
The institute oversees the creation, promulgation, and use of thousands of norms and guidelines that directly impact businesses in nearly every sector including healthcare.
http://www.ansi.org

ELINCS – EHR-Lab Interoperability and Connectivity Specification
ELINCS standardizes the formatting and coding of electronic messages exchanged between clinical laboratories and ambulatory electronic health record (EHR) systems. www.elincs.org

HITSP – Health Information Technology Standards Panel
This is a cooperative partnership between the public and private sectors. The panel was formed for the purpose of harmonizing and integrating standards that meet clinical and business needs for sharing information among organizations and systems.
www.hitsp.org

HL7 – Health Level 7
HL7 provides a comprehensive framework and related standards for the exchange, integration, sharing, and retrieval of electronic health information that supports clinical practice and the management, delivery, and evaluation of health services.
http://www.HL7.org

ICD – International Statistical Classification of Diseases and Related Health Problems
ICD provides codes to classify diseases and a wide variety of signs, symptoms, abnormal findings, complaints, social circumstances, and external causes of injury or disease.
http://www.cms.hhs.gov/ICD9ProviderDiagnosticCodes

LOINC – Logical Observation Identifiers Names and Codes
The purpose of LOINC® is to facilitate the exchange and pooling of clinical results for clinical care, outcomes management, and research by providing a set of universal codes and names to identify laboratory and other clinical observations. http://loinc.org

NCPDP – National Council for Prescription Drug Program
NCPDP creates and promotes the transfer of data related to medications, supplies, and services within the health care system through the development of standards and industry guidance.
http://www.ncpdp.org

Figure 8-6: Examples of Standards Setting, Certifying, and Supporting Organizations

NIST – National Institute of Standards and Technology

NIST is the federal technology agency that works with industry to develop and apply technology, measurements, and standards. NIST is also the organization responsible for leading the development of the core health IT testing infrastructure that will provide a scalable, multi-partner, automated, remote capability for current and future testing needs. http://www.nist.gov and http://healthcare.nist.gov/testing_infrastructure/index.html

OMG – Object Management Group

An international, open membership, not-for-profit computer industry consortium. OMG Task Forces develop enterprise integration standards for a wide range of technologies and an even wider range of industries. http://www.omg.org

SNOMED-CT – Systematized Nomenclature of Medicine – Clinical Terms

A comprehensive, multilingual clinical healthcare terminology coding system supported by the International Health Terminology Standards Development Organization (IHTSD), an international not-for-profit organization based in Denmark. http://www.ihtsdo.org/snomed-ct

Examples of Certifying and Accrediting Organizations

CCHIT – Certification Commission for Health Information Technology

An independent, 501(c)3 nonprofit organization recognized as a certification body for electronic health records. http://www.cchit.org

EHNAC – Electronic Healthcare Network Accreditation Commission

EHNAC's accreditation services help electronic health networks, payer networks, financial services firms, and e-prescribing and other solution providers improve business processes and expand market opportunities. http://www.ehnac.org

With ARRA HITECH certification ruling, new additional certifying organizations are expected to be major players in the future.

Figure 8-6: *Continued*

Professional Organizations that Provide Services Supporting the Deployment of Standards

CORE – Committee on Operating Rules for Exchange

The Council for Affordable Quality Healthcare (CAQH) supports CORE which develops operating rules that direct implementation and use of primarily financial and business administrative data across all stakeholders including providers, clearinghouses, and payers. http://www.caqh.org/benefits.php

IHE – Integrating the Healthcare Enterprise

IHE is an initiative by healthcare professionals and industry to improve the way computer systems in healthcare share information. http://www.ihe.net

Figure 8-6: *Continued*

Standard	Description
Clinical Documentation	
HL7	Health Level Seven International (HL7) is a not-for-profit, ANSI-accredited standards developing organization dedicated to providing a comprehensive framework and related standards for the exchange, integration, sharing, and retrieval of electronic health information that supports clinical practice and the management, delivery, and evaluation of health services. Version 2.x is widely deployed, but due to its constraints with interoperability will be replaced with Version 3.0.[6]
CDA	CDA is the Clinical Document Architecture, an ANSI-certified standard from Health Level Seven (HL7). CDA specifies the syntax and supplies a framework for specifying the full semantics of a clinical document. A CDA can contain any type of clinical content. Typical CDA documents would be a Discharge Summary, Imaging Report, Admission & Physical, Pathology Report, and so on. CDA uses XML, although it allows for a non-XML body (pdf, Word, jpg, and so on) for simple implementations.[7]

Table 8-1: Example Health IT Data and Messaging Standards

Standard	Description
CCD	CCD is the Continuity of Care Document and is a further refinement of the HL7 Clinical Document Architecture (CDA) standard. The CDA specifies that the content of the document consists of a mandatory textual part (which enables human interpretation of the document), and it includes optional structured parts (for system software processing). The structured part is based on the HL7 Reference Information Model (RIM) and provides a framework for referring to concepts from coding systems, such as from SNOMED and LOINC.
	The patient summary contains a core data set of the most relevant administrative, demographic, and clinical information about a patient's healthcare, covering one or more healthcare encounters.
	The CCD specification contains U.S.-specific requirements; its use is therefore limited to the U.S. HITSP selected the CCD as one of its standards.
CCR	The CCR, the Continuity of Care Record, is a snapshot in time of a patient's healthcare, a core data set that shows the most relevant facts about a patient's health status and the physician's treatment of that patient. Like a doctor's handwritten notes, the CCR is prepared by a practitioner at the conclusion of a healthcare encounter.[8] While still in use in a wide variety of settings today, the trend for the industry is moving toward the CCD standard mentioned earlier.
Imaging	
DICOM	DICOM, Digital Imaging and Communications in Medicine, is a global Information Technology standard that is used in virtually all hospitals worldwide to store, print and exchange medical images and derived structured documents as well as to manage related workflow.[9]

Table 8-1: *Continued*

Standard	Description
Laboratory	
ELINCS	ELINCS is an EHR-Lab Interoperability and Connectivity Specification. It standardizes the format and coding of electronic messages exchanged between clinical laboratories and ambulatory electronic health record (EHR) systems.[10]
LOINC	The Laboratory Logical Observation Identifiers Names and Codes database, LOINC®, is used to facilitate the exchange and pooling of clinical results for clinical care, outcomes management, and research by providing a set of universal codes and names to identify laboratory and other clinical observations. The Regenstrief Institute, Inc., an internationally renowned healthcare and informatics research organization, maintains the LOINC database and supporting documentation.[11]
Medication	
NCPDP	National Council for Prescription Drug Programs issues standards for the exchange of prescription-related information that facilitate online prescribing and other pharmacy-related processes.[12]
Services	
HL7 (OMG)	Object Management Group (OMG)[13] and HL7 (see previous boxes) are collaborating to build a set of standard healthcare-domain software components and service interface standards to promote open interoperability across health provider organizations and products.
Vocabulary	
SNOMED CT	SNOMED CT, the Systematized Nomenclature of Medicine Clinical Terms provides the core general terminology for the electronic health record (EHR) and contains more than 311,000 active concepts with unique meanings and formal logic-based definitions organized into hierarchies.[14]

Table 8-1: *Continued*

Standard	Description
ICD-9 ICD-10	The International Statistical Classification of Diseases and Related Health Problems (ICD), published by the World Health Organization (WHO), provides codes to classify diseases and a wide variety of signs, symptoms, abnormal findings, complaints, social circumstances, and external causes of injury or disease. Under this system, every health condition can be assigned to a unique category and given a code. Note: Currently version 9, known as ICD-9 is in wide use in the United States; however, ICD-10, a much more granular version of the coding structure is expected to fully replace ICD-9 in the near future.
CPT-4 CPT-5	The Current Procedural Terminology (CPT®)—the most widely accepted medical nomenclature used to report medical procedures and services under public and private health insurance programs is published by the American Medical Association (AMA).[15]
Administrative and Financial	
ASC X12 HIPAA Standard Transactions	The Accredited Standards Committee (ASC X12), chartered by the American National Standards Institute in 1979, develops electronic data interchange (EDI) standards and related documents for national and global markets, including insurance and government.[16]
Encryption	
AES-128 AES-192 AES-256	The Advanced Encryption Standard (AES) issued by the National Institute of Standards and Technology is a generally accepted standard for encryption.[17]

Table 8-1: *Continued*

your organization are being implemented correctly. Solid audit processes that are well-implemented help you demonstrate that you are in compliance with all of your policies, as well as with relevant federal and state laws and regulations.

Auditing Capabilities That Enable Organizations to
Hold Accountable Those Who Misuse Data

Accountability

Accountability for the inappropriate access to, or use of, a patient's health data is primarily a governance issue. However, technology can provide the necessary tools, incorporating auditing and active monitoring to enable the organization to track and identify the persons who are responsible for inappropriate access. This information can then be used to hold those persons accountable for their actions.

The Connecting for Health Common Framework[18] provides in-depth information on the relevant technology and standards for implementing a secure technology environment in healthcare.

STRATEGIC TECHNICAL CONSIDERATIONS

There are several additional considerations you need to think about as you develop your technical approach.

Integration Engine

As you plan your technical architecture, keep in mind that standards will be constantly evolving. There will never be one right answer nor will there be, in the foreseeable future, only one version of a universal standard in use. As standards evolve, different organizations will update their systems at different times, almost ensuring that multiple versions will always be in use.

You need to identify those technical approaches that will help you maintain flexibility to meet the varying levels of standards adoption by your participating organizations. One approach would be to try and dictate static standards and versions for all participants. This may work for a short time, but the first time one of your participating organizations upgrades its standards version, the process will break.

A more flexible and scalable approach is to develop a normalized (or "universal") set of standards with which all participating organizations will harmonize. With this approach, each organization operates with a suite of standards appropriate for their needs, but they must commit to participating in the standards harmonization services offered by the HIE if they are to participate in exchanging data through the HIE.

In this model, participants send their data, in their own chosen standard format, to an "integration engine." This integration engine then translates the data from the standards in use at the source to a set of standards that are recognized as "universal" standards for that HIE. The same translation occurs when data are sent from the HIE back to an organization. Typically, the data are routed through the "integration engine." Data that are received by the integration engine that are not in a compatible format with the system in use at the organization requesting information will be translated into the format that the receiving institution can use in their systems. The integration engine approach ensures technical and semantic interoperability across the exchange. Figure 8-7 shows how the integration engine normalizes data across disparate systems.

This harmonization approach is more flexible than attempting to impose static standards system-wide. It is certainly a more efficient approach than one in which each

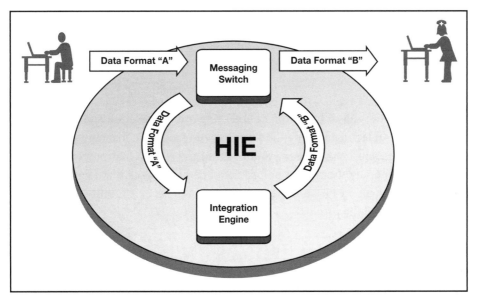

Figure 8-7: The Integration Engine. © 2009 Mosaica Partners, LLC.
Used by permission.

organization is required to map its standards to every other participating organization in a one-to-one mapping approach.

Integration engines typically include software components that can manage messages between multiple systems. Messages can be in multiple forms, such as HL7, CCD, plain text, or Extensible Markup Language (XML), and the engine translates messages from one format to another. We anticipate significant advances in integration engine approaches and the underlying technology in the near future. For example, the Object Management Group, with its Model Driven Message Interoperability (MDMI) standard, has developed an approach where a message format can be published in a software-executable file that can be used by integration engines. When you discuss your technical options with various vendors, make sure to ask them to describe how they handle ensuring interoperability.

Open Source versus Proprietary Products

Another key question you need to address is whether you will use open source or proprietary products. There has been a lot of discussion in the past few years regarding the merits and drawbacks of open source products versus proprietary products. In this section, we will briefly acquaint you with some of each.

The acquisition of open source products is often touted as being virtually free because this software, along with its source code, is readily available on the Internet or from supporting vendors. Proprietary products, on the other hand, like those found in most commercially available applications, contain source code that is protected by intellectual property rights and is typically not disclosed. In the case of proprietary products, you pay the vendors for use of the product and the vendor supports updates and changes. Charges you incur vary by vendor.

Characteristics of Open Source Software

Discussed next are some of the open source specific characteristics. Consider these characteristics as you explore your technical options.

Flexibility

Open source customers have the option of obtaining implementation and maintenance support from several technically qualified vendors or technical consultants. Those who choose to use open source products are not tied to the source that provides the software. Users are generally thought to be protected from the potential "sunset" of software or vendor bankruptcy because there is a broad Internet community of supporters and developers behind the product.

Collaboration

Another major advantage of open source is that it can be optimized through the collaboration of ideas and solutions between the users, developers, and other partners who cooperate to advance the open source software. While each open source software product tends to develop its own user community, other groups, such as commercial vendors, can be used to obtain add-ons and enhancements to the open source software.

Cost

Long-term, open source savings may be substantial since the user is not paying for typical costs associated with commercial products such as marketing, upgrades, and, in some cases, technical support. As mentioned earlier, technical support can often be obtained through the software community. Open source encourages collaboration, enables sharing between applications, and is vendor independent.

> **Caution**
>
> Open source
> software is not free.

Weighing the Pros and Cons

Often, those considering using open source software believe that the software is free, but it is not completely free. While the open source code is free to download, users must still make many of the same investments as one would when purchasing commercial software. This includes the costs associated with installation, training, maintenance, and upgrades.

Open source software does require specific technical expertise, which may be lacking in provider organizations and/or HIEs. This expertise can be obtained from consultants or vendors who specialize in configuring open source software, but it is not necessarily free. You need to consider, however, that once you have customized the software for your needs, you will be responsible for maintaining it. There is little or no economy of scale for support that you would receive from a vendor whose product is operating in multiple locations.

More information on open source for HIEs is located on the HIMSS HIE content website at www.himss.org/ASP/topics_FocusDynamic.asp?faid=141.

SERVICE MODEL FOR TECHNOLOGY

You also need to determine the type of technology service model that you will implement. In the past, most technical services were delivered via the client-server model. In this model there are one or many servers dedicated to providing and managing the application and the data. Historically, this required that at least some part of the application resided on the "client," or the user's computer. Typically, the organizations owned or leased the required hardware and employed in-house staff to manage the system.

With the near ubiquitous use of the Internet today, there are some very different options. Today, many applications are provided as a service over the Internet. The common terms you hear associated with this model are application service provider (ASP) and software as a service (SaaS).

The ASP is the business that provides services to customers over the network. Services may range from access to a single application to access to a growing number of software services. ASPs generally house and support the hardware; many run and support the software application as well.

SaaS uses the ASP model in which the hardware and software are housed in a remote location and supported by a vendor. In SaaS, a vendor licenses its software to a wide variety of users for use on demand. Generally, ongoing fees are established for the use of the services. One major advantage to this model is that it can greatly reduce the amount of up-front capital required for start up, as the amount of hardware needed to be purchased is minimal, and there are various financial options for obtaining the right to use the applications.

We strongly recommend that you consider the SaaS approach as you determine your technology path.

PLANNING AND SELECTING
THE HIE TECHNICAL PLATFORM

Although technology is only an enabler of HIE, it is typically very resource intensive to plan, implement, and operate. It is expensive both from the perspective of required financial outlay and from the hours required to install, learn, operate, and maintain. In this section, we highlight some of the critical components and decisions that you need to consider as you specify and implement your HIE technical capabilities.

Planning and Selecting the Technology Architecture

Once the HIE services you plan to offer are defined and your key governance policies are in place, you are ready to begin to document the specific requirements that will guide your technology selection. The functional requirements and technical specifications you develop are derived from both the business services you plan to provide to your state, region, or community and the policies required to run your HIE.

This stage of your project uses the many well-established best practices found in the existing body of knowledge related to good IT project management. This is a mature field with many excellent resources. Appropriate best practices include understanding which services that the business or HIE will provide, understanding how the participants in the HIE expect to use the system, and what data and computing require-

> **Caution**
>
> Being overly rigid in your technical specifications can add substantially to your costs.

ments are needed for the operational system. These elements, plus many more, will form the foundation of the Request for Proposal (RFP) you will issue when you are finally ready to select your technology. We will not devote much space to a discussion on technology project management here; however, we provide a list of resources at the end of this chapter that you can access for further information.

Document Your Requirements

The first step in determining your technology needs is to define your functional require-

> Using key descriptive use cases is valuable to help you identify your functional requirements.

ments. These requirements are based upon the capabilities that your technology must provide to support the business services that you will offer. Functional requirements are derived from your Business Plan and specify what the technology needs to do to deliver the required services and enforce your organizational policies—and under what circumstances. They also describe the expected performance levels for the system. This first step is critical in determining the type of technology you will implement. We have found that developing and using key descriptive use cases is valuable in helping you identify and document your functional requirements.

Technical specifications describe the behavior of the system and how it will operate on the technical level. They are derived from the functional requirements. In the past, technical specifications were very detailed because systems were built from scratch. In today's environment, you need to develop technical specifications that are only detailed enough to ensure that you provide enough specific guidance to the vendor who is proposing a technology product. You do not need to technically design the entire solution.

Key questions to address in developing your technical specifications include:
- How will you enable the HIE to deliver its services?
- What type of exchange model(s) is appropriate for your community?
- How will you implement your security policies?
- How will you determine unique patient identifiers?
- How will you integrate the data from disparate sources?
- What standards will you use and how will you implement them?
- What parts of the technical infrastructure might you be able to leverage or share from your statewide HIE efforts?
- What is the appropriate infrastructure for interfacing with other HIEs, with your state HIE and with the NHIN?
- What response times are required by the users?
- How will data retrieval and access be managed?
- How much of the technology and technical support will be outsourced—or will you support it all yourself?

Note: Your functional requirements must reflect your specific HIE. As you move into the technical specifications phase, you need to consider the options that various vendors' products provide. You may need to modify some of your specifications so that you can choose a "best-fit" vendor solution. If you are overly rigid in your specifications to the point that no vendor can accommodate your HIE without significant modifications to their product, you run the risk of adding substantially to the amount of money you will spend on your system. That said, do not let a vendor drive you to a system that is not suitable for your community.

Research Technical Options and Vendor Approaches

Once you understand the business requirements and technical specifications, you are ready to move into the technology acquisition phase. Of course, initiating this phase of the project requires you to be aligned with the current state of progress of your other workgroups.

You need to ensure that your organization's governance is at a mature enough point to effectively make decisions. The Business & Financial workgroup needs to be far enough along to ensure that there is available funding to procure the necessary products and provide enough resources for the required ongoing support.

This alignment in timing and maturity is critical to your success. Too many organizations have thought they were ready to acquire technology only to find, late in the process, that their board and/or their stakeholders were not willing or able to make the required investment. Let's assume, however, that you have passed that hurdle and it is time to seriously search for technology.

Vendor Products – Online Buyers' Guide

There are many good resources that provide information on vendors and their associated products and services. One very good resource is the online HIMSS Buyers' Guide,[19] which includes a description of a wide variety of health IT vendors and their products.

The key in using any of the vendor resource listings or tools is that you must have a clear understanding of the technology strategy, technology options, and framework that you will use to support your business and service model. This provides the HIE strong technical direction in meeting its needs and will prevent "drift" into vendor-proposed solutions that may not be appropriate. These tools can help you learn about the different vendors' approaches and the technical solutions available to support your HIE and guide you to vendors that may be appropriate for you.

SELECT THE VENDOR(S)

Unfortunately, there is no one right technology approach for all HIEs. Your choice of technology depends upon your particular needs. Vendors offer a variety of choices—from component products to "complete" HIE solutions. You need to decide what is best for your organization. Do you want to work with just a single vendor? Alternatively, do you want the flexibility to work with more vendors and integrate their products? There are pros and cons to each approach.

The RFP Process

Once you fully understand your requirements, your approach, and the supporting technology that is available, it is time to create an RFP for your technology. It is important for you to select the right technology solutions that will support your policies, your service offerings, and your stakeholder needs. An RFP is used to invite vendors to submit a proposal to address your specific needs.

Use your functional requirements and your technical specifications to create your RFP. As mentioned earlier, an RFP must be specific enough to convey a sufficient amount of information on what you require so that vendors can respond appropriately. However, it should not be so stringent that you leave vendors no room to use their expertise to propose innovative approaches. Remember, you are looking for the most advantageous approach/product for your organization. It is the vendors' job to propose the technical solution.

A good RFP process is structured and focused on determining the best vendor for your project. The RFP is a written description of your project requirements. It includes a description of the background of the project and of your organization and the goals you want to achieve. In addition to your functional requirements and technical specifications, you should include a description of the terms you want to be included in the future contract. The RFP and the chosen vendor proposal should form the basis of the contract you subsequently negotiate with the vendor.

Make sure you provide specific instructions to the vendors on how to get their questions answered, whom they should contact, and how they should respond to the proposal. Specifically define what should be included in their response and the criteria for your decision making. Remember that you are using this as a tool to find the best product(s) for your organization. Providing as much detail as you can without over-specifying the product will save you time and aggravation when you evaluate the proposals you receive. Figure 8-8 lists the essential components for an RFP.

1. **Administrative Information** – Provide information in this section, such as the name of your organization, contact information, and significant dates for the RFP process.
2. **Background** – Provide a description of your organization and the project in general. This provides prospective vendors with a good understanding of your situation.
3. **Instructions** – Provide information as to how the vendor should respond to the RFP, how to submit questions, where to send the proposal, formatting and other relevant information for responding to the RFP.
4. **Project Requirements** – Specifically describe what you are seeking. It should include your functional requirements and relevant technical specifications including standards for interoperability and any relevant certifications you require of the product or the vendor. It should also include any constraints placed upon the vendors. Make sure you explicitly state your security requirements and request that the vendor provide a detailed description of how patient privacy is maintained.
5. **Cost Proposal** – Provide the framework for how you want the vendor to respond regarding their proposed costs. It can be in the form of a spreadsheet or other table. You may request details such as a breakdown in the costs of procuring the

---

1. Administrative Information

2. Background of organization and the project

3. Instructions to vendors

4. Project requirements and vendor response

5. Cost proposal

6. Vendor profile information

7. Vendor references

8. Terms of contract

Figure 8-8: Essential Components of a Good RFP

technology, implementation costs, ongoing maintenance fees, and consulting fees. It is also a good practice to request that the vendor provide a detailed estimate of any other costs you might incur that are not directly related to this vendor's fees.

6. **Vendor Profile Information** – Request detailed information from the vendor about their company, such as length of time in business, number of employees, and financial stability.

7. **Vendor References** – Be specific in asking for reference sites that reflect the same, or at least similar, requirements as your HIE. There are many variations in the services provided by HIEs, and it is important to find vendors that are providing services similar to those you expect to provide. The references provided will then be able to give you an accurate description of their satisfaction relating to your needs and may also advise you of situations that you should take into account when contracting.

8. **Terms of Contract** – This is especially important in the public sector wherein contracts must follow a strict protocol, and the conditions must be transparent; however, it is also useful for private organizations to help set contract expectations.

Decision Criteria

As you create your RFP, you should develop your decision criteria tool as well. This tool is typically a weighted list, based on the degree of importance, of the elements you are asking the vendors to address. There is no one right way to develop this list. The content of the list and the weighting depends upon your specific requirements. Use your business requirements and technical specifications as the basis for building your evaluation criteria.

Remember, various vendors have strengths in different areas. It is in your best interest to decide what is most important to your organization. Having objective criteria upon which to make your vendor selection is an invaluable tool as you analyze the various proposals you receive. Figure 8-9 provides example criteria you may want to include in your tool. These are just some examples. The type of product and the delivery method the vendor proposes will impact the criteria you use to evaluate the offering.

- Amount of initial investment required to acquire the technology
- Ongoing costs required to maintain and upgrade the product
- Specific functionality that you (a) require or (b) desire
- Cost of installation/implementation
- Amount of vendor-supplied support for implementation and ongoing operations
- Number of current customers using the product that you are considering
- Vendor references
- User training and support—cost, quantity, and content
- Technical training and support—cost, quantity, and content
- Additional features the vendors includes and any associated costs
- Price
- Terms of payment

Figure 8-9: Example Vendor Selection Criteria

According to Gina Perez, Executive Director of Delaware Health Information Network (DHIN), in their efforts to evaluate vendors, not only did DHIN write an RFP and hold demonstrations, they provided test scripts and scenarios for the vendors to demonstrate. Some of these test scripts included specific errors to determine how the products would handle errors.

Figure 8-10 summarizes the steps we have discussed that you need to consider as you select your technology vendor.

Who Needs to Be Involved

Representatives from the technical workgroup will be valuable subject matter experts as you move through the RFP process—from vendor identification, evaluation, and selection through contract negotiation. However, the process should be led by the executive director who has the authority to negotiate the contract. Make sure to keep the board informed of progress, as they are responsible for approving the funding. Figure 8-11 provides tips for negotiating a vendor contract.

Figure 8-12 lists key objectives we discussed in this chapter that you need to complete as you design, procure and implement your HIE technical platform.

DEVELOP/ASSEMBLE, IMPLEMENT, AND TEST THE TECHNOLOGY

At this point you will have identified and obtained the appropriate resources for the technical implementation of your HIE. It is the responsibility of your technology project manager to manage the entire technology implementation and testing phases of the project, including the work of the vendor. Remember, this is your project and it needs to align with your business requirements and meet your expectations. Your project manager may have the day-to-day responsibilities for managing this portion of the project, but the executive director and the board are accountable.

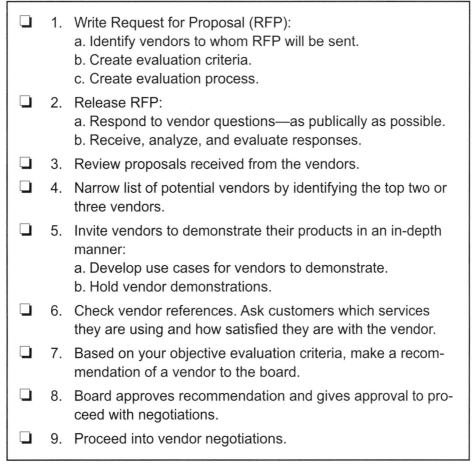

Figure 8-10: Checklist—Selecting the Vendor

- Talk with other HIEs to learn from their experience in dealing with specific vendors.
- Link progress payments to the vendor meeting agreed-upon performance milestones and acceptance criteria.
- Include as much vendor support service as possible in the base price. Beware of added costs for support and installation.
- Include service level agreements (SLAs) in your contract negotiations. These contractually bind the vendor and ensure that the HIE timeline and stakeholder expectations are met.
- Review the contract closely to make sure there are no hidden fees and that your best interests are being served.

Figure 8-11: Tips for Negotiating a Vendor Contract

It is beyond the scope of this book to include all of the steps for technology implementation and testing. Figure 8-13 provides a high-level checklist of key activities to consider.

❑   1. Develop functional requirements documentation.
❑   2. Develop technical specifications documentation.
❑   3. Research technical options and vendors.
❑   4. Research technical security tools.
❑   5. Research the marketplace.
❑   6. Select vendor.
❑   7. Implement and test the technology.

Figure 8-12: Checklist—Planning for and Selecting the Technology

❑   1. Determine the appropriate technical service model.
❑   2. Acquire, lease, or contract for technology or services.
❑   3. Create (technology) implementation plan.
❑   4. Create plan to prepare participant sites for technical connection.
❑   5. Develop security test plan.
❑   6. Develop quality assurance plan and metrics.
❑   7. Create performance metrics and measurement process.
❑   8. Create capacity management plan and metrics.
❑   9. Create overall test plan – including scenarios and use cases.
❑   10. Identify risks to implementation and develop mitigation approaches.
❑   11. Install technical components.
❑   12. Perform initial test of technical components.
❑   13. Modify implementation as required by test results.

Figure 8-13: Checklist—Installing and Testing the Technology

As a review, Figure 8-14 provides a recap many of the steps you should include as you develop your technical platform.

CHAPTER SUMMARY

In this chapter we used the typical services provided by an HIE as a basis to discuss the various components of the technical implementation. Security, since it is vital to the HIE's success, was integrated into the discussion of the services that the technology needs to support.

We discussed the importance of technical interoperability and provided examples of the various technical standards in use—and being developed—today.

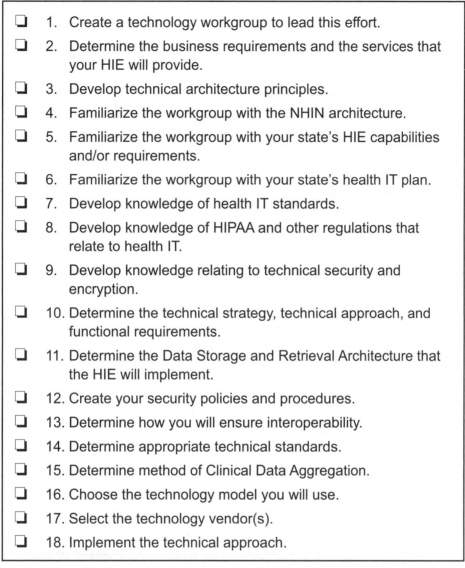

❏   1. Create a technology workgroup to lead this effort.

❏   2. Determine the business requirements and the services that your HIE will provide.

❏   3. Develop technical architecture principles.

❏   4. Familiarize the workgroup with the NHIN architecture.

❏   5. Familiarize the workgroup with your state's HIE capabilities and/or requirements.

❏   6. Familiarize the workgroup with your state's health IT plan.

❏   7. Develop knowledge of health IT standards.

❏   8. Develop knowledge of HIPAA and other regulations that relate to health IT.

❏   9. Develop knowledge relating to technical security and encryption.

❏ 10. Determine the technical strategy, technical approach, and functional requirements.

❏ 11. Determine the Data Storage and Retrieval Architecture that the HIE will implement.

❏ 12. Create your security policies and procedures.

❏ 13. Determine how you will ensure interoperability.

❏ 14. Determine appropriate technical standards.

❏ 15. Determine method of Clinical Data Aggregation.

❏ 16. Choose the technology model you will use.

❏ 17. Select the technology vendor(s).

❏ 18. Implement the technical approach.

Figure 8-14: Checklist—Creating the HIE Technical Platform

We also took you through the steps of identifying the right technical models and approaches for your HIE. We provided guidance on the steps you need to take to acquire and implement the technical solution that is optimal for your HIE.

This phase of your project is complete when the technology is operating, it has been satisfactorily tested, and you can demonstrate that it is performing as required. You are now ready, from a technology standpoint, to begin your pilot. In Chapter 9, *Becoming Operational*, we discuss running the pilot and moving into the operational stage.

CASE STUDIES

CareSpark

Liesa Jenkins, Executive Director, CareSpark

As mentioned earlier, CareSpark decided early on to build their HIE based on standards. They use a document-based architecture to share information with participants. If a participant is not able to use ("consume") a CCD document, CareSpark will store the record in their own clinical data repository for potential future use. They maintain a registry of all documents available for a patient.

Services offered by CareSpark include:

- Central MPI
- Document locator
- Interface engine
- Document repository
- Translator to CCD
- Consent management (Master Patient Options Preference)

The Master Patient Options Preference (MPOP) consent manager is a custom-built engine that tracks patient consent. This tool is used by both the provider and HIE to ensure they are complying with the patient's level of consent. While each provider is responsible for gaining the patient's consent to share their data with the exchange, CareSpark uses the MPOP as an additional check to determine whether to accept or reject any record sent to them. For example, if a record is sent to them and they do not show that there is consent to share the information, they will reject the records relating to that patient until the patient consent is confirmed.

New Mexico Health Information Collaborative (NMHIC)

Jeff Blair, Director of Health Informatics, LCF Research

NMHIC uses a Federated Architecture that enables clinician access to patient information from edge servers located at each providers' facility. While the administrative/clinical information is stored at the edge server, patient demographic information is stored in the Master Person Index (MPI), which is centrally located at LCF Research. When an authorized clinician has patient consent to access that patient's information from NMHIC, the clinician will locate that patient in the MPI and then the centralized Record Locator Service (RLS) will access that patient's records from each of the provider edge servers where that patient has previously received care. A Summary Patient Record will then be displayed on the NMHIC Web portal for review by the authorized clinician. An audit record is kept of every clinician access to every patient's information.

The architecture deploys an instance of an edge server database and interface engine on a server behind the firewall of each healthcare provider organization. The edge server receives data from each facility's existing administrative and clinical information systems. These data flow into and are then permanently stored on the organization's edge server. For additional information on the NMHIC technical architecture, please see New Mexico State HIE Strategic and Operational Plan.[20]

Michigan Health Information Network (MiHIN)
Technical Guiding Principles

Beth Nagel, Health Information Technology Coordinator, Michigan Department of Community Health

Following is an overview of the MiHIN Technology Guiding Principles.[21] They include statements about how the MiHIN must behave to fit into the existing business and technical environment. One of the initial decisions made within their Technical Workgroup was that the MiHIN would be designed to be an open, scalable, and extensible infrastructure. The guiding principles were revisited and tested several times during workgroup discussions, debates, and the various perspectives considered in the design. The guiding principles acknowledge that MiHIN will:

- Be built from numerous vendor products which must interoperate.
- Be vendor agnostic.
- Support multiple communication protocols within reason (FTP, SOAP, Sockets, etc.).
- Be a hybrid architecture that will not be entirely federated or centralized.
- Comply with the latest interoperability standards but be practical enough to get something working.
- Undertake an incremental approach to implementing a statewide architecture.
- Be consistent with national industry standards (Web services, etc.).
- Focus on designing information exchange, not end-user applications.
- Interoperate with existing state government systems like public health surveillance and reporting.
- Use Web services for real-time communications where feasible.
- Interoperate with sub-state HIEs.
- Interoperate with the NHIN.
- Be highly secure and Health Information Portability and Accountability Act (HIPAA)-compliant for all external communication paths.
- Maintain the privacy of patient data.
- Be extensible (capable of adding new functions or services easily).
- Be scalable (capable of adding more users, transactions, other volumes of work easily).
- Support delegated user authorization, authentication and administration.
- Support auditing.
- Be able to support data and analytical capabilities.
- Be cost effective to maintain.

RESOURCES

Department of Health & Human Services. AHRQ Health IT Adoption Toolbox. http://healthit.ahrq.gov/portal/server.pt?open=512&objID=1135&mode=2&pid=DA_986270&cid=DA_986503&p_path=/DA_986503&pos=#Answer. Accessed April, 2010.

Technical Architecture Frameworks

EHRS Blue Print. Canada Infoway. An Interoperable EHR Framework, CanadaHealth Info April, 2006. http://knowledge.infoway-inforoute.ca/EHRSRA/doc/EHRS-Blueprint-v2-Exec-Overview.pdf. Accessed November, 2009.

Connecting for Health Common Framework, 2006. The Common Framework helps health information networks share information among their members and nationwide while protecting privacy and allowing for local autonomy and innovation. It consists of a set of 17 mutually-reinforcing technical documents and specifications, testing interfaces, code, privacy and security policies, and model contract language. Markle Foundation. Connecting for Health Common Framework, 2006. http://www.connectingforhealth. org/commonframework/#guide. Accessed November, 2009.

Federal Health Architecture. The Federal Health Architecture (FHA) charter is to bring federal agencies together to improve efficiency and effectiveness in government health IT operations. Department of Health & Human Services. Federal Health Architecture. http://www.hhs.gov/fedhealtharch/. Accessed November, 2009.

NHIN CONNECT. CONNECT is a software solution that is the universal on-ramp for federal agencies, allowing federal agencies to securely link their existing systems to the NHIN. More than 20 federal agencies collaborated to build CONNECT through the Federal Health Architecture (FHA).

Nationwide Health Information Network (NHIN): Prototype Architectures.
In its first year, the NHIN established four consortia to design and evaluate standards-based prototype architectures for the NHIN.
http://healthit.hhs.gov/portal/server.pt?open=512&objID=1190&parentname=CommunityPage& parentid=1&mode=2&in_hi_userid=10741&cached=true. Accessed November, 2009.

New York SHIN. NY Statewide Health Information Network for New York
(SHIN-NY) Technical Architecture Overview V1.0, November 3, 2008. http://www.nyehealth.org/files/ File_Repository16/pdf/SHIN-NY_TechArch_20081125.pdf. Accessed November, 2009.

Other Resources

The State HIE Cooperative Agreement Program. The State HIE Cooperative Agreement Program has been given the charge to develop or facilitate the creation of a technical infrastructure that supports HIE services. According to the State HIE Collaborative Grant, these services include:
- Electronic eligibility and claims transactions
- Electronic prescribing and refill requests
- Electronic clinical laboratory ordering and results delivery
- Electronic public health reporting (i.e., immunizations, notifiable laboratory results)
- Quality reporting
- Prescription fill status and/or medication fill history
- Clinical summary exchange for care coordination and patient engagement

http://healthit.hhs.gov/portal/server.pt?open=512&objID=1336&mode=2&cached=true. Accessed November, 2009.

CalRHIO. CalRHIO Safety Net Health Information Exchange Toolkit. HIE Program: Technology Procurement. http://www.calrhio.org/?cridx=412. Accessed November, 2009.

HIMSS. HIMSS Health Information Exchange Open Source Task Force. Exploring the Use of Open Source Software for Health Information Exchange, A White Paper. Posted July, 2009. http://www.himss.org/ content/files/HIEOpen%20SourceWhitePaper071709.pdf. Accessed November, 2009.

HIMSS. HIMSS Health Information Exchange Open Source Task Force. Exploring the Use of Open Source Software for Health Information Exchange, A White Paper. Posted June, 2008. http://www.himss.org/content/files/HIE_FY08_Open_Source.pdf. Accessed November, 2009.

CalRHIO. Safety Net Health Information Exchange Toolkit. http://www.calrhio.org/?cridx=410. Accessed November, 2009.

Techsoup (the technology place for non-profits). The RFP Process: An Overview. Posted May 10, 2006. http://www.techsoup.org/learningcenter/techplan/page5507.cfm. Accessed November, 2009.

The following resources are provided by the Agency for Healthcare Research and Quality (AHRQ) of the U.S. Department of Health & Human Services.

AHRQ Health IT Adoption Toolkit. Introduction to Public Domain and Open Source Software. http://healthit.ahrq.gov/portal/server.pt?open=512&objID=1135&mode=2&pid=DA_1015012&cid=DA_986406&p_path=/DA_986294/DA_1015012/DA_986406&pos=#Answer. Accessed November, 2009.

AHRQ Health IT Adoption Toolkit. What are the Relevant Standards for Health IT? http://healthit.ahrq.gov/portal/server.pt?open=512&objID=1135&mode=2&pid=DA_1003217&cid=DA_986400&p_path=/DA_986294/DA_1003217/DA_986400&pos=#Answer. Accessed November, 2009.

AHRQ Health IT Adoption Toolkit. Which are the Key Standards Organizations?

http://healthit.ahrq.gov/portal/server.pt?open=512&objID=1135&mode=2&pid=DA_1003217&cid=DA_986397&p_path=/DA_986294/DA_1003217/DA_986397&pos=#Answer. Accessed November, 2009.

Department of Health & Human Services. AHRQ Health IT Adoption Toolkit, Planning for Technology Implementation. http://healthit.ahrq.gov/portal/server.pt?open=512&objID=1135&mode=2&pid=DA_986294&cid=DA_1014962&p_path=/DA_986294. Accessed November, 2009.

REFERENCES

1. HIMSS Patient Identity Workgroup. Patient Identity Integrity. Posted December, 2009. http://www.himss.org/content/files/PrivacySecurity/PIIWhitePaper.pdf. Accessed April, 2010.

2. The text from the 1998 Omnibus Appropriations Act (not the official title) signed into law (PL 105-277): "SEC. 516. None of the funds made available in this Act may be used to promulgate or adopt any final standard under section 1173(b) of the Social Security Act (42 U.S.C. 1320d-2(b)) providing for, or providing for the assignment of, a unique health identifier for an individual (except in an individual's capacity as an employer or a health care provider), until legislation is enacted specifically approving the standard."

3. IHE International. Profiles. http://www.ihe.net/profiles/. Accessed April, 2010.

4. HIMSS Annual Connect-a-Thon 2010. http://www.himss.org/ASP/ContentRedirector.asp?ContentId=73001&type=HIMSSNewsItem. Accessed October, 2010.

5. HIMSS. *HIMSS Dictionary of Healthcare Information Technology Terms, Acronyms and Organizations, Second Edition.* Chicago: HIMSS; 2010.

6. Health Level Seven International (HL7). About HL7. http://www.hl7.org/about/index.cfm. Accessed April, 2010.

7. Health Level Seven International (HL7). CDA FAQ. http://www.hl7.org/documentcenter/public/faq/cda.cfm. Accessed April, 2010.

8. ASTM International. ASTM E2369 - 05e1 Standard Specification for Continuity of Care Record (CCR). http://www.astm.org/Standards/E2369.htm. Accessed April, 2010.

9. Digital Imaging and Communications in Medicine (DICOM). Strategic Document. Posted March 30, 2009. http://medical.nema.org/dicom/geninfo/Strategy.pdf. Accessed April, 2010.

10. California Health Care Foundation. What Is ELINCS? http://elincs.chcf.org/. Accessed April, 2010.

11. Logical Observation Identifiers Names and Codes (LOINC). History, Purpose, and Scope. http://loinc.org/background. Accessed April, 2010.

12. National Council for Prescription Drug Programs (NCPDP). Standards. http://www.ncpdp.org/standards.aspx. Accessed April, 2010.

13. Object Management Group (OMG). Joint Development Effort by OMG and HL7 Leads to Initiation of Two New Healthcare SOA Standards. Posted January 22, 2007. http://www.omg.org/news/releases/pr2007/01-22-07.htm. Accessed April, 2010.

14. Health Terminology Standards Development Organisation. About SNOMED CT. http://www.ihtsdo.org/snomed-ct/snomed-ct0/. Accessed April, 2010.

15. American Medical Association (AMA). American Medical Association House of Delegates 2009 Interim Meeting Handbook Plus Addendum. http://www.ama-assn.org/ama1/pub/upload/mm/38/i-09-complete-handbook-addendum.pdf. Accessed April, 2010.

16. Accredited Standard Committee (ASC X12). About ASC X12. http://www.x12.org/. Accessed April, 2010.

17. National Institute of Standards and Technology (NIST). The XTS-AES Validation System (XTSVS). Posted March 31, 2010. http://csrc.nist.gov/groups/STM/cavp/documents/aes/XTSVS.pdf. Accessed April, 2010.

18. Markle Foundation. Connecting for Health. http://www.connectingforhealth.org/commonframework/#guide. Accessed April, 2010.

19. HIMSS On-Line Buyer's Guide. http://onlinebuyersguide.himss.org/. Accessed October, 2010.

20. New Mexico State HIE Strategic and Operational Plan. www.nmhic.org. Accessed October, 2010.

21. State of Michigan MiHIN Shared Services Strategic Plan. http://www.michigan.gov/documents/mihin/MiHIN_Shared_Services_Strategic_Plan_4-30-10_320156_7.pdf. Accessed October, 2010.

CHAPTER 9

Becoming Operational

*People will remember a good start and will forgive you later
if you make mistakes. But they never forget a bad start.*

Dick Thompson
Executive Director/CEO
Quality Health Network

INTRODUCTION

The objective of this chapter is to help you transition from the formation stage to the operational stage. In this chapter, we pull together all of the work you have done so far and address what else you need to do to move into the operational stage. In prior chapters, we laid out the path to develop the various components of the HIE. This chapter discusses how you integrate those components to prepare for, and move into, your operational stage. The pieces all come together in your implementation and operations plans.

As we have often said throughout this book, there is no one right way to form a health information exchange. It is especially true as you enter the operations stage. There is an element of art to weaving all of the component capabilities you have developed and then transitioning those to the operational stage. This transition is done in phases, not all at once.

Your work now is to assemble the components into an integrated whole. Later, once you are operational, you will begin to optimize your HIE's operations as you learn more of what it takes to meet your stakeholders' needs and the needs of your community. These will be continuously moving targets, and you need to ensure you can adequately respond to, and adapt to, your constantly changing environment. To be successful and sustainable, you must become an adaptive organization.

It is at this point in the journey that you transition from the project plan that was used to form your HIE—and develop your initial set of capabilities and services—to the Operational Plan, which will guide you as you begin to operate and grow the organization. The Implementation Plan is the bridge that takes you from the formation stage to actual operations.

We begin this chapter with a recap, by domain, of the capabilities you should have built so far and what you should have accomplished. We then discuss what you still need to do in each of those domains to transition to the operational stage. We also discuss how you need to weave all of these components into an integrated, complete operating environment. Don't worry if your efforts have not been perfect. You are definitely further along the journey than when you started!

RECAP OF ACTIVITY BY DOMAIN
Stakeholder Engagement & Participation

In the Stakeholder Engagement & Participation domain, you built your initial communication plan. You have implemented many components of your Stakeholder Engagement Plan and included stakeholders every step of the way. That effort is critical and helps to ensure active participation in your operational stage. You have learned to communicate effectively with your stakeholders, determined their wants and needs and incorporated their input into all of your planning, so that the governance and business models are ones in which they *want* to participate. You continue that effort now as you recruit additional stakeholders to participate in your pilot and become participating members of your operational HIE.

Later, in the section on *Developing Your Capabilities and Implementation Plan*, we discuss how what you have learned about your stakeholders will be instrumental in integrating the component capabilities you developed into your Operational Plan. You will use your early Communication and Stakeholder Engagements Plans as the basis for your Marketing Plan. The Marketing Plan—a logical extension of the communication plan—is focused on making people aware of your services, aware of the benefit of using those services, and letting them know that you are now "open for business."

Of course, stakeholder engagement and participation efforts do not end here. This is only the beginning of a continuous and long-running dialogue with your stakeholders. Enjoy the continuing conversation.

Governance

By now you should have a formal governance structure in place. You developed your core principles—and your policies are a reflection of those principles. You have established your governing board and may even be an independent legal entity. You have paid close attention to the legal requirements for the protection of patients' right to privacy of their health information, and this is directly reflected in your privacy policies and your security policies and procedures.

Your board understands their role and accepts the responsibilities and accountabilities associated with their role in running the organization. Fiduciary and governance roles are well documented and the processes you use to govern your organization, including financial accountability, membership requirements, and voting rights have been established, are in use, and are open and transparent.

Here we discuss how to use the organizational policies and procedures you have developed and put in place to develop your operational procedures. Depending upon the governance model you have adopted, the majority of the work involved in developing your operational structure and policies may fall to the executive director and HIE staff—to prepare and submit to the board to approve—or, your board may be more active and directly involved in developing these policies and procedures.

Also in the section on *Developing Your Capabilities and Implementation Plan*, we discuss what you need to do to ensure that the appropriate operational policies, procedures, and processes are in place to help you move smoothly into operation. These operational policies and procedures will encompass all aspects of your operation and use input from the stakeholder participation, business, and technical workgroups. These groups should continue working together closely and should coordinate their efforts as you move into operations.

Business & Finance

In Chapter 5, *Creating Your Strategic Plan*, and Chapter 6, *Your Business Plan Defines How Delivering Value Drives Your Sustainability*, we showed you what you needed to do to develop your Strategic and Business Plans and to focus these plans on delivering value to your stakeholders. Assuming that you followed our advice in this book, you have involved your stakeholders directly in developing your plans, so you should have a funding model that aligns with your stakeholders' wants and needs and is consistent with your organization's requirements for sustainability. In this chapter, we discuss what you need to do to turn your plan into a reality.

Earlier, in Chapter 7, *Protecting Patient Privacy*, we discussed the necessity of implementing Business Associate Agreements (BAAs) to maintain compliance with HIPAA regulations and the HITECH Act. These agreements will be executed with each of the participants in your HIE.

Working with input from the Stakeholder Engagement & Participation, Governance, Privacy, and Technical & Security workgroups, you also need to develop participation agreements for those organizations planning to use your services. These agreements spell out the mutual expectations for service by the HIE participants and the financial remuneration you will receive for providing those services.

One key component of the participation agreements is the Service Level Agreement (SLA). The SLA addresses the specifics of the services that you provide, such as a description of the service; under what conditions it is provided; the metrics indicating successful delivery; and the penalties, if any, for failure to meet the defined service levels. As with all contracts and agreements, you should seek legal advice to ensure that you are operating within all relevant laws and regulations.

Privacy

As previously emphasized, the protection of a patient's privacy is paramount. It is an essential subset of your overall organizational governance. The various requirements related to protecting a person's health information underpin many of the policies and procedures to which your organization is obligated to adhere. You have sought out (and hopefully heeded) legal advice as you developed these policies. You have considered not only the statutory and regulatory landscape to develop your policies and procedures but have also incorporated the nuances specific to your community that were identified by the efforts of the Stakeholder Engagement & Participation workgroup.

Now, as you anticipate the exchange of real patient health information, you are ready to create the operational policies and procedures to ensure that patient privacy is properly protected. This effort requires that your Privacy workgroup works closely with the security experts from the Technology & Security workgroup. Ensure that the security tools and processes align with your organizational policies and that they are implemented appropriately. The security policies and procedures that you developed are also reflected in the BAAs and the participation agreements developed by the Business & Finance workgroup.

You have used the "5 A's" of Security to guide the creation of your privacy policies. Your security policies and procedures have been researched and developed to complement your privacy policies.

Technology & Security

You have invested significant amounts of time and resources in defining your technical approach and platform and acquiring and implementing the technical infrastructure components necessary to enable the electronic exchange of health information. Your technical infrastructure was designed and developed to serve the mission of your HIE: to provide the services that your stakeholders require—in the way they need them; to provide appropriate access to information; to prevent inappropriate access to patient data; and to ensure that data are not lost or corrupted. You have acquired, implemented, and tested the necessary technology and tools to ensure that you can support the safe and secure exchange of data.

In this chapter, we discuss the remaining steps you will need to undertake to transition your tested infrastructure into a well-managed operational environment. Since the field of technology implementation is mature, and there is an abundance of resources to assist you with developing your technical implementation plan, we do not go into detail on that subject in this chapter.

DEVELOPING YOUR CAPABILITIES AND IMPLEMENTATION PLAN

Throughout the formation stage you have developed stakeholder relationships; governance and business knowledge, skills, and capabilities; appropriate privacy policies; security policies and procedures; and technology tools and competencies to launch your HIE. However, no two transitions into operations are the same. Many things, including your stakeholder wants and needs, your board decisions, your financial resources, and your environmental practicalities will influence your transition. It is worth noting that this is a time when your board responsibilities may also change as you move from the formation stage to the operational stage. The role of the board will typically evolve from one of hands-on management to more of an oversight and governance role.

Your Implementation/Roll out Plan consolidates all of these components and describes how you will transition the services and capabilities that you developed in the formation stage into an operational HIE.

As mentioned previously, you have developed capabilities in all of the five domain areas: Stakeholder Engagement & Participation, Governance, Business & Finance, Privacy, and Technology & Security. Table 9-1 provides an example of how the capabilities you built in these areas will translate to operations. It shows, by domain, some of the initiatives that we have discussed in the previous chapters, the organizational capabilities that you developed by completing the initiatives, and the resulting preoperational activities you need to complete to ensure you are prepared for full operations.

STAKEHOLDER AND COMMUNITY PARTICIPATION

By now, if you have followed the leading practices related to stakeholder engagement and participation, your key stakeholders and the community at large will be well informed on your efforts and, by and large, supportive. Do not let them down now.

You are asking them to actually implement the changes that you have been talking about and toward which you and they have been working. Continual two-way communication remains critical to your success. Continue to reach out and listen to your stakeholders and keep them informed as you finalize your implementation plans. Be mindful of any pockets of resistance and work diligently to listen to and address any concerns you hear.

Your community needs to be able to trust the HIE with the handling of its personal health information.

User Training and Support

A key to the success of your HIE is that you must provide services that integrate with your providers' normal work processes. This means that your users, who you should think of as your customers, must be well-trained and well-supported in using the HIE's services. We believe that good user training provides the necessary foundation that leads to success for those using your services. Nothing can replace the value of time spent, early in the adoption of your HIE services, for

> Your community needs to be able to trust the HIE with the handling of their personal health information.

training and supporting your users in how to use the system properly and making them comfortable. If end users feel comfortable and are successful in using your services, they will tell their colleagues and recommend to them that they also participate. If they don't feel successful, they will also tell their colleagues.

One danger of inadequate preparation and training of users is that if they are not successful early on with the HIE, they are likely to become disenchanted and fatigued. As a result, they may discontinue using the HIE. There is strong evidence of this happening at many individual provider practices that have tried to implement an EMR system without adequate preparation and support.

Our experience shows that your users should be actively involved in developing the training plan so that it suits their needs and is relevant to their work. Your training plan activity began with the initial assessment of your provider community and concludes with the successful use of your services by your "customers." It must also be able to address new customers. Figure 9-1 provides a checklist to use during the development of your Training Plan.

Domain	Initiatives Undertaken	Capabilities Developed	Preoperations Activities
Stakeholder Engagement & Participation	• Develop Stakeholder Engagement Plan • Develop and implement Communication Plan	• Build and maintain stakeholder participation • Provide information to, and receive input from, stakeholders	• Develop training • Develop end-user support • Develop ongoing communication
Governance	• Develop organizational principles • Create decision-making process • Determine membership criteria	• Develop policies to run the organization according to its mission and core principles	• Develop processes to efficiently provide operational services in a manner aligned with organizational principles and policies
Business & Finance	• Create Strategic Plan including vision, mission, objectives, and strategies • Develop funding model	• Manage the organization according to your mission and principles • Provide sufficient revenue to sustain (and grow) the organization	Develop and implement: • Business associate agreements • Participation contracts • Service level agreements • Charging model(s) and processes • Management process for revenue stream(s)

Table 9-1: Example of Activities Necessary for Operational Readiness

Domain	Initiatives Undertaken	Capabilities Developed	Preoperations Activities
Privacy	• Develop policies to protect a patient's right to privacy • Develop processes to ensure organization is always in compliance with all applicable laws and regulations	• Provide stakeholder confidence in the confidentiality of the data	Implement: • Security processes • Policy implementation procedures
Technology & Security	• Determine technical approach • Develop technical architecture • Acquire technology • Implement technical components	• Exchange electronic health information using a secure, reliable technical infrastructure	Develop and implement: • Operational systems procedures • Technical support processes • End-user support processes • Technology maintenance processes • Security procedures

Table 9-1: *Continued*

❏   1. Develop training plan:
        • Assess and understand end-user needs.
        • Set training goals.
        • Determine training delivery methods.
        • Create a training program.

❏   2. Develop and document new work process flows that incorporate routine data sharing with the HIE.

❏   3. Develop training materials.

❏   4. Procure and schedule training sites and facilities.

❏   5. Train the trainers.

❏   6. Enroll and schedule users for training.

❏   7. Hold the training session(s).

❏   8. Evaluate effectiveness of the training session(s) through feedback and monitoring the types of questions and support calls you encounter.

❏   9. Make changes to the training as required.

❏   10. Provide follow-up training sessions and provide reinforcement as needed.

Figure 9-1: Checklist—Training Plan Development

Whom to Involve

You should involve people with a background in designing adult education; people who can map (and revise) clinical workflows; those who understand how your system will work; those with documentation skills; people who can perform the education; and those who can organize and schedule the actual training sessions. Remember to use your State Designated Entity and Regional Extension Center as potential sources for assisting you with your training programs.

Help Desk and Support Resources

Ensure that the end-user support processes are tightly linked to both the training function and the technical function. Training and technology administrators should be informed of excessive requests for specific "How do I?" types of queries, so that the answers to these questions can be incorporated into future training sessions. Problem reports should be grouped and classified to identify areas in which the system may need repair or updating by the technology group or vendor. The technical group should keep the help desk informed, in advance, of any changes made to the system and then provide advice on how to address user questions about the changes. This requires an ongoing dialogue and coordination within your organization.

BUSINESS AND OPERATIONS MANAGEMENT

In this section, we discuss how the governance you have developed—along with the policies and procedures—is used to create the foundation for operational management.

> Your operational management structure and governance are the tangible implementation of the organization's mission, principles, and governance into a practical customer-facing reality.

Prepare the Team for Operations

Your operational management structure and governance provide the framework within which your HIE will operate. This operational management structure and governance is the tangible implementation of the organization's vision, mission, principles, and governance into a practical, customer-facing reality.

While you generally will want to have a full set of approved organization-level policies created before you begin to work on your operational policies and procedures, it is possible to create some operational policies and procedures before all of the organizational policies are finalized. However, it is important to remember that your operational policies and procedures must align with your organizational policies. Figure 9-2 provides a list of activities to consider as you develop your operational management and governance.

When complete, these activities provide a written set of approved operating principles, policies, and procedures—governance—for business, finance, and technical operations. You will also have documented operational roles and responsibilities.

❏   1.   Create your operating principles.

❏   2.   Develop operating policies and procedures.

❏   3.   Approve operational policies and procedures.

❏   4.   Develop and implement operational processes to ensure implementation of policies and procedures.

❏   5.   Ensure required agreements are in place with partners.

❏   6.   Define operational roles and responsibilities.

❏   7.   Develop operational budget.

❏   8.   Develop operational metrics.

Figure 9-2: Checklist—Operating Structure

Participant Agreements Signed

As with the signing of the BAAs, successfully executing participant agreements is dependent upon having involved your stakeholders all along the journey. Continue to dialogue with your stakeholders as you develop your participation agreements. Key steps in developing and negotiating your participation agreements are found in Figure 9-3.

1. Ensure that you have sufficient operating policies, procedures, and management to ensure a secure, smooth ongoing exchange of information.

2. Discuss data sharing individually with the appropriate personnel of each of the targeted participants to obtain input as you develop your participation contract.

3. Obtain legal advice on the contracting process as needed.

4. Create your participation contract.

5. Ensure that the HIE has the procedures in place to monitor and meet all service-level requirements that are specified in the contract.

6. Work with each participant to address any issues with the contract.

7. Gain agreement from providers to send data through the HIE, according to their contract terms.

8. Work with each participant organization to get contracts signed.

9. Ensure that each stakeholder who signs a participation contract also has signed a Business Associate Agreement.

Figure 9-3: Key Components of the Participation Agreement

Whom to Involve

Include people who understand how to operate and run the business, finance, and technical aspects of an organization. Also, include someone knowledgeable in the area of defining organizational roles and responsibilities. Most HIE organizations have a relatively small staff. In many organizations, there are between four and six people on staff. Tap your community or other external resources to help with this effort.

TECHNICAL OPERATIONS PLAN

Your Technical Operations Plan includes developing and implementing the policies and procedures for running and supporting the technical platform, the technical support of end users, the technical support for the infrastructure of the participating organizations, and the implementation of your security procedures and tools. The specifics of the plan may vary depending upon the technical service model you have chosen, but the components should all be included.

Develop the help desk processes and end-user support tools with input from the Stakeholder Engagement & Participation workgroup. This will help ensure that you develop operational processes and acquire tools that make the end-users' experience with the HIE as smooth, efficient, and "painless" as possible.

Figure 9-4 contains a checklist of key areas you should make sure you address in your Technical Operations Plan.

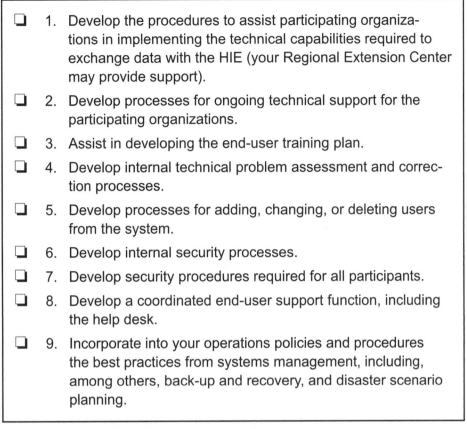

❏ 1. Develop the procedures to assist participating organizations in implementing the technical capabilities required to exchange data with the HIE (your Regional Extension Center may provide support).

❏ 2. Develop processes for ongoing technical support for the participating organizations.

❏ 3. Assist in developing the end-user training plan.

❏ 4. Develop internal technical problem assessment and correction processes.

❏ 5. Develop processes for adding, changing, or deleting users from the system.

❏ 6. Develop internal security processes.

❏ 7. Develop security procedures required for all participants.

❏ 8. Develop a coordinated end-user support function, including the help desk.

❏ 9. Incorporate into your operations policies and procedures the best practices from systems management, including, among others, back-up and recovery, and disaster scenario planning.

Figure 9-4: Checklist—Technology Infrastructure

You will also need to develop an approach to reconcile stakeholder demands for service and the realities of your budget and capabilities to deliver on those demands or expectations. Work with the Business & Finance workgroup to ensure that the SLAs align with your delivery capabilities. Set realistic expectations and communicate them as appropriate.

THE PILOT

The pilot phase is both the final step of your formation phase and the first step in the operations phase; it is the transition point. The pilot is a trial implementation of your HIE. Many consider the pilot as the "soft opening." It validates that you have all the right components in place for daily operations and that they integrate smoothly. Its successful completion marks the point at which you are ready to move into the operational phase.

Many times a pilot is associated only with the technical environment. However, if done properly, the pilot phase encompasses much more than just testing the technology. It includes testing your governance, your policies, and your decision making. You will also validate that your Stakeholder Participation Plans and your Business and Financial Plans are scalable and realistic. In other words, a good pilot is a preoperational test of *all* of your business processes—including your technology infrastructure.

The pilot phase involves successfully testing the integration of your:

- Stakeholder Engagement and Participation Plan
- Training Plan
- On-boarding Plan—describes the order in which participants will be added and the processes to be used
- Technology Implementation Plan
- Privacy Procedures
- Revenue and Financing Plan
- Operational Management
- Implementation Plan—site and community
- Operations Launch Plan
- User Support and Help Desk

Figure 9-5: Components of the Pilot

Your implementation pilot is the final testing of your integrated processes and systems prior to the HIE going live. This is when all of the components you have developed in the formation stage come together for fine-tuning, before you open your operations to the broader community. Expect to make some minor modifications and address some problems; however, by this point all the components should already be fully tested and functional. The pilot is the opportunity to run your system in a real, but limited, environment. Typically, you will be exchanging real patient data among real HIE participants but on a small scale.

The difference between pilot and full-scale operations is that a pilot involves only a small subset of your intended operational participants. However, the pilot should reflect your intended operational environment in all other ways. Figure 9-5 lists a summary of components essential for the pilot.

The purpose of the pilot is to identify and resolve any problems or issues that may occur in an integrated operations environment that have not been previously identified through component testing—also known in IT project management parlance as unit testing. Running the pilot on a small scale keeps any negative effects to a small (and hopefully flexible) representative population and provides you the opportunity to correct any problems before expanding to a more widespread operational environment.

As you have been doing throughout the formation stage, you will again go back to your mission statement and core principles to ensure that you have put in place the capabilities required to achieve your mission in a way that is consistent with your vision, mission, principles, and stakeholder needs.

There are many steps involved in running a good pilot. These are summarized in Figure 9-6.

A successful pilot means that you have all the necessary components in place, that they are working together well, and that you are ready for larger-scale operations. A successful pilot provides tangible evidence that you have developed and implemented the capabilities required to exchange healthcare information.

❏ 1. Develop key performance indicators/critical success factors (KPIs/CSFs) and metrics for the pilot. To fully evaluate your pilot, it is critical that you have metrics in place so that you can identify problems and issues and correct them.

❏ 2. Choose your pilot participants carefully and make sure that they fully understand the implications of being involved in a pilot. This includes the knowledge that problems may arise and that this is not yet a production environment. Choose participants who are willing to work with you to identify and correct any problems. Make sure that they know to expect glitches and that you are fully prepared to work with them to correct any problems they encounter.

❏ 3. Develop a process to identify and address issues and to correct problems that arise during the pilot phase.

❏ 4. Work collaboratively with the technical teams of the participating organizations that will be exchanging data in the pilot to assist them in preparing their technical environment.

❏ 5. Work with the pilot organizations to complete business associate and participation agreements with your HIE before they participate in the pilot.

❏ 6. Implement the pilot and maintain metrics on its operation.

❏ 7. Make necessary modifications to address issues.

❏ 8. Continue the pilot phase until all issues are addressed and you are confident that you have the capability to efficiently and securely exchange data, meet your defined metrics, and deliver on the SLAs.

❏ 9. Publicize the success of the pilot exchange.

❏ 10. Begin final preparations for becoming operational.

Figure 9-6: Checklist—Pilot Activities

IMPLEMENTATION AND ROLLOUT PLAN

The Implementation Plan provides the roadmap for understanding which organizations will be added as participants to the HIE and in which order they will be added. It is developed jointly with your stakeholders and lends credibility and predictability to the expansion of your HIE. The plan includes the schedule for user preparation and training; timing for technology set-up; estimation of staffing needs; and your overall path to full operations. One advantage to a good Implementation Plan is that it shows that the organization has the discipline to take the initiative to identify possible risks and develop activities and processes to address and mitigate those risks and issues.

❏   1. Develop and implement operational policies and procedures.

❏   2. Develop and implement financial control for operations.

❏   3. Develop and implement quality assurance policies and procedures.

❏   4. Develop procedures for assisting participants to modify existing, or implement new, workflow processes that include using shared patient information. Your Regional Extension Center is a good resource to work with on this effort.

❏   5. Develop and implement end-user training for using the HIE.

❏   6. Develop the end-user support plan—including a help desk.

❏   7. Develop metrics and the processes necessary for measuring and reporting on your performance.

❏   8. Conduct the pilot and identify and correct any problems.

❏   9. Develop and implement processes to identify and correct problems that arise once you are in the operations stage.

❏   10. Preload patient data into the system to ensure that the HIE is useful from the beginning.

❏   11. Implement the "Go Live" phase of your Communication Plan. This includes:
   • Communicating with the community and stakeholders about the services that will be provided.
   • Developing and delivering marketing messages and materials for the "grand opening."
   • Conducting a "soft opening" prior to the full community opening.
   • Fostering ongoing communication with the local press to assure widespread coverage of the implementation.

❏   12. Obtain approval from the board for officially moving to the operational stage.

❏   13. Announce the beginning of official operations and the "grand opening."

Figure 9-7: Checklist—Components of Implementation Plan

You can begin planning your implementation prior to the time when you have a clear idea of your go-live date. Don't wait until your pilot is completed. This is the culmination of your formation-related project planning. You know you are ready when:

- Your stakeholders are engaged and willing to participate.
- You have commitments to exchange data.
- Your governance is in place and operating effectively.
- Your privacy policies are developed.
- Your security policies and procedures are in place.
- Your business plan is ready and participants agree with your revenue model.
- Your technical capabilities are ready.
- You understand the state of readiness of your various stakeholders.
- Your pilot is considered successful.

Successful implementation is dependent upon the close coordination and alignment among all the team members and continuous interaction with your stakeholders. Document your expectations for the implementation and ensure that you have defined the processes and measurements to gauge your progress. Make sure to publicize your progress. To achieve these objectives and be fully prepared to move to the operational stage, there are several key steps to include in your implementation plan. Figure 9-7 provides an example of a final checklist of the components that you need to include in your Implementation/Roll-out plan.

BEGIN INITIAL OPERATIONS

You are now ready to open for business! It is important to have a designated point in time to become operational and then to publicize it. Consider publicizing and hosting a community event to launch the operational HIE.

Once you are officially operational, your obligations as a Business Associate are now the same, under HIPAA, as a *covered entity* and you are now legally responsible for ensuring that all the appropriate policies, procedures, and audit capabilities are in place. Becoming operational means that all prerequisite activities and milestones for the establishment of an HIE have been met and you have enough providers participating to make the exchange meaningful.

The second phase of your journey is just beginning. You have laid the foundation and developed the capabilities, which will move you down the path to improving healthcare in your community and beyond!

CHAPTER SUMMARY

In this chapter, we have provided a recap, by domain, of the capabilities you developed during the Formation Stage. We then described the activities/initiatives you needed to complete in order to become operational, including developing operational policies and procedures, developing training and support capabilities, and creating and executing participation agreements.

We discussed the pilot and how this is an implementation trial with a small set of participants. It is used to fully test the integrated capabilities and services that will constitute your operational environment.

Lastly, we discussed the importance of the Implementation Plan and how a good plan will provide clarity and predictability as you ramp up your operations.

Once you complete the activities of this chapter, you will have an operational HIE.

> *Forming a Health Information Exchange is a journey.*
> *This book provides you with the right tools and points you in the right direction.*
> *But only you, and your stakeholders, can take the actual steps*
> *necessary to successfully form and operate an HIE.*
>
> CONGRATULATIONS! Remember to CELEBRATE YOUR SUCCESS!

CASE STUDIES
HealthInfoNet Principles of Operation[1]

- Information privacy and security is the highest priority.
- Information is organized and presented to promote effective clinical decision making and patient safety.
- Access to individually identified health information is based on the formal consent of the individual.
- Access to individually identified health information for the purpose of promoting public health and safety is based on established state and federal law.
- Participation in the system is open to and affordable for all individual health providers involved in the care of a patient.
- Participation in the system is voluntary and includes the right of any individual or organization to withdraw from participation.

Guiding Principles & Common Values of the Quality Health Network, Grand Junction, Colorado[2]

- Improve health of residents, efficiencies, and satisfaction of providers and patients.
- Maintain patient privacy and security. Create QHN as trusted third party.
- Health information technology is a common cost and enabler—sharable among participants.
- Patient information exists to improve health outcomes—not to be used as a competitive tool for individual stakeholders.
- Participants are to direct as much content as possible into the network to drive usage.
- Promote Quality Health Network as the preferred delivery system of patient information for all EMRs.
- Provide resources to maintain the network, train and support users, and facilitate quality improvement efforts until the network can sustain itself.
- Promote use of e-prescribing tools to update shared patient info in Quality Health Network databases.
- Combine relevant resources in order to:
  - Prevent unnecessary duplication and fragmentation of medical data

- Promote interoperability of systems
- Promote opportunities to cost-share
- Establish common standards for:
  - Best practices of care
  - Information exchange
  - Privacy and security
- Promote equitable treatment for all to reduce commonly absorbed costs associated with treatment of the underserved populations.
- Promote Quality Health Network business model among all participants.

RESOURCES

Department of Health & Human Services. AHRQ Health IT Adoption Toolkit, Planning for Technology Implementation. http://healthit.ahrq.gov/portal/server.pt?open=512&objID=1135&mode=2&pid=DA_986294&cid=DA_1014962&p_path=/DA_986294. Accessed April, 2010.

Department of Health & Human Services. Consumer Education and Engagement. http://healthit.hhs.gov/portal/server.pt?open=512&objID=1280&PageID=16051&mode=2&cached=true. Accessed October, 2010.

TechRepublic. Shinder, Deb. Plan Your End-User Training Strategy Before Software Roll-Out. Posted March 6, 2006. http://articles.techrepublic.com.com/5100-10878_11-6045557.html. Accessed April, 2010.

Department of Health & Human Services. Health Information Security & Privacy Collaboration (HISPC). Provider Education Toolkit (PET) Explained. Posted June 9, 2009. http://healthit.hhs.gov/portal/server.pt/gateway/PTARGS_0_10741_875062_0_0_18/PET_Workshop.pdf. Accessed November, 2009.

Department of Health & Human Services. Health Information Security & Privacy Collaboration (HISPC). (2009, June 09). Provider Education Toolkit (PET). Posted June 9, 2009. http://www.secure4health.org/. Accessed November, 2009.

eHealth4NY.org. Resources. http://www.ehealth4ny.org/resources.html. Accessed April, 2010.

Department of Health & Human Services. AHRQ Health IT Adoption Toolkit, Planning for Technology Implementation. http://healthit.ahrq.gov/portal/server.pt?open=512&objID=1135&mode=2&pid=DA_986294&cid=DA_1014962&p_path=/DA_986294. Accessed April, 2010.

CareSpark (2008). Evaluation Plan 2007 - 2011. Posted 2008. http://healthit.hhs.gov/portal/server.pt/gateway/PTARGS_0_10731_865204_0_0_18/CareSpark%20evaluation%20plan%202007-2011%20v2.pdf. Accessed April, 2010.

REFERENCES

1. Interview with Devore Culver on April 19, 2010.
2. Provided by Dick Thompson, Executive Director/CEO, Quality Health Network.

Example Mission and Vision Statements

CareSpark

Mission

Improve the health of people in NE Tennessee and SW Virginia through the collaborative use of health information.

Delaware Health Information Network

Vision

The vision of DHIN is to develop a network to exchange real-time clinical information among all health care providers (office practices, community clinics, hospitals, laboratories and diagnostic facilities, etc.) across the state to improve patient outcomes and patient-provider relationships, while reducing service duplication and the rate of increase in health care spending.

Mission

To develop a community-based health information network to facilitate communication of patient clinical and financial information, designed to:
- Promote more efficient and effective communication among multiple health care providers, including, but not limited to, hospitals, physicians, payers, employers, pharmacies, laboratories and other health care entities;
- Create efficiencies in health care costs by eliminating redundancy in data capture and storage and reducing administrative, billing and data collection costs;
- Create the ability to monitor community health status; and
- Provide reliable information to health care consumers and purchasers regarding the quality and cost-effectiveness of health care, health plans and health care providers.

Goals

The DHIN's five primary goals serve as the basis for interoperability among all healthcare providers in the state of Delaware:
- To improve the care received by patients served by Delaware's health care system and to reduce medical errors associated with the often inaccurate and incomplete information available to providers of medical care.

- To reduce the time required and financial burdens of exchanging health information among health care providers and payers (necessary for patient care), by addressing the currently siloed and unintegrated model of distribution methods and dramatically increasing use of electronic means.
- To improve communication among healthcare providers and their patients to provide the right care at the right time based on the best available information.
- To reduce the number of duplicative tests to afford specialists a more comprehensive view of the patient upon referral from his/her primary physician and to expedite the reporting of consultant opinions and tests/treatments between specialists and the referring physicians.
- To improve the efficiency and value of electronic health records (EHR) in the physician office and to assist those physicians without an EHR to better organize and retrieve test results.

HealthBridge

Mission

Our mission is to improve the quality and efficiency of healthcare in our community. To do this, we serve as a trusted third party working with all participating healthcare stakeholders to facilitate creation of an integrated and interoperable community healthcare system.

HealthInfoNet

Mission

Develop, promote, and sustain an integrated, secure, and reliable regional information network dedicated to delivering authorized, rapid access to person-specific healthcare data across points of care that will support
- Improved patient safety
- Enhanced quality of clinical care
- Increased clinical and administrative efficiency
- Reduced duplication of services
- Enhanced identification of threats to public health
- Expanded consumer access to their own personal health care information

Principles of Operation

- Information privacy and security is the highest priority.
- Information is organized and presented to promote effective clinical decision making and patient safety.
- Access to individually identified health information is based on the formal consent of the individual.
- Access to individually identified health information for the purpose of promoting public health and safety is based on established state and federal law.
- Participation in the system is open to and affordable for all individual health providers involved in the care of a patient.

- Participation in the system is voluntary and includes the right of any individual or organization to withdraw from participation.

MedVirginia

Vision

[We envision] Central Virginia to be one of the most electronically integrated communities of healthcare providers in the country.

Mission

To organize, coordinate and serve provider interests in health care information technology by providing a system for community-wide clinical information exchange that enables improved clinical workflow and the attainment of "meaningful use" of health IT. MedVirginia also helps providers utilize health IT to create and maintain patient-centered medical homes for those they serve.

New Mexico Health Information Collaborative (NMHIC)

Mission

To improve healthcare quality and efficiency through the creation of a statewide health information exchange network that is trusted and valued by all stakeholders (employees/patients, employers, physicians, health systems and health plans).

North Carolina Healthcare Information and Communications Alliance, Inc. (NCHICA)

Vision

NCHICA will be a leader in the drive for innovative applications of IT to improve healthcare in North Carolina and the nation.

Mission

To improve health and care in North Carolina by accelerating the adoption of information technology and enabling policies.

Pennsylvania eHealth Initiative

Mission

The mission of the corporation is to: (a) Enable the use of information technology to improve healthcare quality and efficiency and ensure patient safety for all Pennsylvanians; (b) Ensure secure, confidential access to health information to enable individuals and communities to make the best possible health decisions.

Rochester RHIO, Rochester, NY

Mission

The mission of the Rochester RHIO is to provide the Rochester medical service area with a system for a secure health information exchange that allows for timely access to clinical information and improved decision making. The primary goal is to share timely and accurate patient healthcare information in a secure environment to improve patient care.

Workgroup Charter Template and Examples of Charter Contents

Workgroup Charter Template

An HIE domain charter represents the mutual consent and commitments of the workgroup relating to:
- Desired outcomes
- Scope of activities
- Concept of operations
- Resources and skills required
- Responsibilities and authorities
- Communication and coordination
- Schedule of activities and work products

Each domain workgroup should prepare its charter and consult the charters of the other domain workgroups before starting its own work. Charters address the scope, sequence, and content of work in each of the five principal HIE formation domains:
- Stakeholder Engagement & Participation
- Governance
- Business & Finance
- Privacy
- Technology & Security

An effective charter has five main sections of content. A charter's level of detail depends on the complexity of the desired work products and the size of the domain team. However, the following are important elements on which the workgroup should agree, at least implicitly but better explicitly. A fully developed charter contains the following five sections:

Administration

- Formal workgroup name (name used in documents and within HIE formation community)
- Purpose of workgroup (domain description and reason team exists)
- Charter effective date and duration of workgroup activities
- Designated workgroup leader (single point of contact and decision maker)
- Workgroup roster with contact information and roles (e.g., core member, advisor)
- Accountabilities (identified external person to whom workgroup is accountable)

- Communication plan (within workgroup, to other workgroups, to Executive Team, to public)
- Signatures of workgroup members affirming mutual consent and commitment

Inputs (What We Need to Do Our Work)

- Workgroup authorities (ability to spend funds, commit HIE, make decisions)
- Workgroup resources on which goals are based (skills, information, facilities, external support)
- Evaluation of significant risks to workgroup operations and delivery of work products
- Risk management strategies and contingencies (e.g., resources, skills, funding required)
- Required technology (e.g., online workspace for collaboration or as document repository)

Process (How We Will Work)

- Scope of activities
- Workgroup operations concept
- Decision making process (e.g., consensus, majority, executive)
- Conflict resolution and problem solving principles and practices
- Processes to change membership or leadership as workgroup evolves
- Meeting processes (frequency of meetings, attendance policies, contingencies)
- Documentation processes (e.g., work products, charter modifications)

Output (What We Will Produce)

- Performance objectives (specific deliverables, dates and performance measurements)
- Deliverables approach (how work products will be prepared and delivered)

Outcomes (What We Will Accomplish)

- Performance evaluation (criteria, procedure to determine when quality of work is sufficient)
- Delivery of final work products

Depending on the size of the HIE formation effort, the complexity of the environment and length of time required, the charter development effort may result in a large document. If appropriate, the workgroup may prepare an executive summary for day-to-day guidance and communication of workgroup principles and commitments internal to the HIE formation effort and to external stakeholders.

Example Contents of Workgroup Charters

Although each workgroup charter will address all of the elements in Appendix B, some elements are more important than others to the success of the respective HIE formation domains. In developing their charters, each workgroup may require considerable discussion to understand and agree on the scope, resources and activities needed to fully contribute to the success of the HIE formation.

For example, the charter section entitled "Process: Scope of Activities" describes the workgroup tasks necessary to establish the infrastructure and operations of the domain. This scope differs across domains and may well differ across HIEs, depending on the intended nature of the HIE and needs of the local community. The following is an illustrative description of typical scope of activities for each of the five domains, to be discussed and adapted as appropriate and consistent with the direction from the HIE Executive Team.

Example Stakeholder Engagement & Participation Workgroup Charter Scope of Activities

The mission of the Stakeholder Engagement & Participation Workgroup is to understand stakeholder wants and needs and design sustainable mechanisms to optimize stakeholder engagement in the HIE. As a critical part of the engagement process, this workgroup develops and helps implement a communication plan. Common activities include:

- Assess the community to identify key stakeholders to involve in the HIE planning efforts.
- Define and confirm stakeholder wants and needs related to healthcare and an HIE.
- Assess the current state of the community regarding awareness of HIE.
- Identify community barriers to HIE and recommend strategies to address barriers.
- Develop, implement and advise operation of an HIE communications strategy and plan.
- Work with the Business & Finance Workgroup to develop HIE value propositions.
- Work with the Privacy Workgroup to accommodate stakeholder privacy concerns.

Example Governance Workgroup Charter Scope of Activities

The mission of the Governance Workgroup is to establish the legal and governing structures of the HIE. This workgroup sets expectations and defines policies, roles and responsibilities, decision making, and accountability. Common activities include:

- Determine and recommend an appropriate formal governance model.
- Develop and recommend organizational principles, policies and procedures.
- Define and recommend organizational/board roles and responsibilities.
- Develop and recommend decision-making process for the HIE governance.
- Establish principles and practices of financial oversight.
- Draft and obtain approval for the Business Associate Agreements.
- Draft and obtain approval for participant agreements.
- Develop and recommend a process to evaluate HIE operational performance.
- Develop and recommend a process to review mission and strategic direction.
- Identify and approve a Board of Directors.

- Draft organizational bylaws.
- Advise the HIE on approaches to obtain formal legal status.
- Work with the Business & Finance Workgroup to integrate management and governance.

Example Business & Finance Workgroup Charter Scope of Activities

The mission of the Business & Finance Workgroup is to develop a sustainable economic model and executable business plan for the HIE. This group will create the business model that is the basis for creating sustainability for the HIE. Common activities include:

- Articulate and document value propositions for key stakeholder segments.
- Develop and recommend a revenue model and pricing structure for HIE services.
- Develop and recommend a three-year pro-forma capital and operating budget.
- Recommend a funding plan, including coordination with the local business community.
- Recommend contracting and business relationship principles.
- Develop and recommend a management model and business plan.
- Identify the risks of the HIE business plan and recommend mitigation strategies.
- Design and recommend financial management principles and systems.
- Work with the Governance Workgroup to integrate management and governance.

Example Privacy Workgroup Charter Scope of Activities

The mission of the Privacy Workgroup is to develop policies, procedures, and practices to ensure protection of a patient's health information. The group is responsible for ensuring that the policies meet all applicable state and federal regulations. This group will also educate the HIE governing board regarding their roles and responsibilities in protecting a patient's privacy. This group will also serve as advisors to the technical architecture group to ensure alignment between privacy requirements and the associated technical security implementation. Common activities include:

- Understand local, state and federal laws and regulations concerning privacy.
- Establish a working relationship with the State Designated Entity (SDE) or other privacy groups as appropriate.
- Articulate and recommend privacy requirements relating to the acquisition, handling and exchange of health information for the HIE.
- Develop and recommend privacy policies in the following areas:
  - Authorization
  - Authentication
  - Access
  - Audit
  - Accountability
- Recommend roles and responsibilities relating to protecting health information.
- Educate the broader HIE formation team regarding privacy and security.

- Work with the Stakeholder Engagement & Participation Workgroup to develop and communicate messages regarding privacy.
- Work with the Technology & Security Workgroup to ensure alignment between the privacy policies and the security implementation.
- Work with the Governance Workgroup to integrate the privacy policies into the organization.

Example Technology & Security Workgroup Charter Scope of Activities

The mission of the Technology and Security Workgroup is to develop an approach for, and design, the technical architecture for the HIE. The technical architecture includes the hardware, software, applications, data, network, security protocols and standards that will be used to develop the technical and security capabilities of the HIE.

This workgroup will also be responsible for recommending and implementing the products that will be purchased/developed for the operation of the HIE. Common activities include:

- Understand national efforts relating to HIE—specifically the work of the NHIN, HITSP, and HISPC projects.
- Develop a thorough understanding of the HIT technology marketplace.
- Recommend a technical architecture that meets and supports the HIE business requirements, conforms to national standards and privacy needs, and enables the HIE policies.
- Establish a process to identify, evaluate and recommend technology vendors.
- Evaluate and recommend an appropriate vendor(s) to implement the architecture.
- Design and recommend ongoing technology investments and management practices to ensure sustainable HIE technology performance.
- Oversee the implementation of the technical environment to ensure the HIE is technically ready for operations.
- Work with the Privacy Workgroup to ensure stakeholder privacy concerns and safeguards can be managed within the technology infrastructure and operations.

Rigorous charter development is complementary to creating a business plan and pays significant dividends later in the HIE formation process. Workgroups benefit from considering each charter as an integrated whole, ensuring that each element is consistent with and supports the other elements. For example, desired outcomes must relate to proposed activities and the identified resources required must support those activities.

An experienced HIE charter facilitator can ensure each group creates a charter that is consistent both internally as well as across workgroups. A well-drafted charter lets the workgroup start its activities sooner and reduces the risk later in the formation process of conflict with other workgroups or rework due to inadequate workgroup planning.

Appendix C

Glossary

This glossary provides explanations for key terms, phrases, and acronyms used in Health Information Exchange and in this book. Some terms may have other common definitions when used in other contexts.

Access controls: Hardware, software, or policies that control access to data by controlling access to facilities, networks, computer devices, computer applications, and programs.

Agency for Healthcare Research and Quality (AHRQ): A federal agency of the U.S. Department of Health & Human Services, whose mission is to improve the quality, safety, efficiency, and effectiveness of healthcare for all Americans. Information from AHRQ's research helps people make better-informed decisions and improve the quality of healthcare services. AHRQ was formerly known as the Agency for Health Care Policy and Research. http://www.ahrq.gov/

Aggregated data: A set of data compiled for research, trending, marketing, and the like; because it is "aggregated," information is not identifiable down to the individual health record (identified or de-identified).

American Health Information Community (AHIC): A federal body, chartered in 2005 and formed by the Secretary of the U.S. Department of Health & Human Services to make recommendations to the Secretary on how to accelerate the development and adoption of health information technology. www.hhs.gov/healthit/community/background/

American Health Information Management Association (AHIMA): A professional organization of health information management professionals who work on a wide range of issues, including electronic health record implementation; implementing ICD-10 coding standards; and contributing toward the formation of the Nationwide Health Information Network (NHIN). AHIMA offers a wide range of health information management tools. www.ahima.org

American Medical Informatics Association (AMIA): A professional organization that promotes the effective organization, analysis, management, and use of information in healthcare in support of patient care, public health, teaching, research, administration, and related policy. AMIA performs work, including research, into the development of a policy framework for secondary uses of data. AMIA collaborated with the American Telemedicine Association to form the Health Technology Consumer Council. www.amia.org

American National Standards Institute (ANSI): A 501(c)3 private, not-for-profit organization that oversees the creation, promulgation, and use of thousands of norms and guidelines that directly impact businesses in nearly every sector, including healthcare. ANSI has recently formed the Healthcare Information Technology Standards Panel (HITSP), which will work with the Office of the National Coordinator for Health Information Technology (ONC) on activities to date and the "breakthrough areas" that are under consideration by AHIC. The panel was formed to facilitate the harmonization of consensus-based standards necessary to enable the widespread interoperability of healthcare information in the United States. www.ansi.org

American Telemedicine Association (ATA): A non-profit organization that promotes access to medical care for consumers and health professionals via telecommunications technology. www.atmeda.org

Audit logs: Electronic identifiers generated by hardware (network servers, firewalls, etc.) or software (electronic health records, databases, claims processing systems, etc.) that are used to track the time that data are created, accessed, modified, destroyed, transmitted, and so forth, and identify the individual or entity responsible for the action.

Authentication: (1) A method or methods employed to prove that the persons or entities accessing information are who they say they are. (2) Security measure, such as the use of digital signatures, to establish the validity of a transmission, message, or originator, or a means of verifying an individual's authorization to receive specific categories of information. The process of proving that a user or system is really who or what it claims to be. It protects against the fraudulent use of a system, or the fraudulent transmission of information."[1]

Authorization: A system established to grant access to generally confidential information. Authorization also establishes the level of access an individual or entity has to a data set and includes a management component—an individual or individuals must be designated to authorize access and manage access once access is approved.

Business associate: An agent of a healthcare organization, generally with access to individually identifiable health information, who assists the healthcare organization in conducting business. This definition derives from business associate as defined in the Health Insurance Portability and Accountability Act (HIPAA) Security and Privacy Rules; the term is defined at 45 C.F.R. § 160.103.[2]

Business practices: Organizational practices that are implemented to address the needs of the business in meeting organizational goals; meeting legal requirements; meeting the needs of customers (in healthcare, patients, and health plan members) and remaining profitable.

Centers for Medicare & Medicaid Services (CMS): Federal agency of the U.S. Department of Health & Human Services that is responsible for the administration of the Medicare and Medicaid programs. http://www.cms.gov/

Certification Commission for Healthcare Information Technology (CCHIT): A 501(c)3 non-profit organization recognized as a certification body for electronic health records. It began as joint initiative of AHIMA and the Healthcare Information and Management Systems Society (HIMSS). CCHIT certifies health information technology (HIT) products and has published standards to meet their certification criteria. www.cchit.org

Chief Information Officer (CIO): Job title commonly given to the most senior executive in an enterprise responsible for the information technology and computer systems that support enterprise goals. The CIO typically reports to the chief executive officer, chief operations officer, or chief financial officer.

Chief Information Security Officer (CISO): The senior-level executive within an organization responsible for establishing and maintaining the enterprise vision, strategy and program to ensure information assets are adequately protected. The CISO directs staff in identifying, developing, implementing and maintaining processes across the organization to reduce information and information technology (IT) risks, respond to incidents, establish appropriate standards and controls, and direct the establishment and implementation of policies and procedures. The CISO is also usually responsible for information-related compliance.

Consumer: An end-user of healthcare services. The term can include patients, health plan members, or personal representatives of the patient or health plan member. It can also denote an organization formed to address consumer needs and protect consumer rights.

Contract: A legal instrument that defines a relationship between two or more individuals or entities. It may define working relationships; legal requirements; or deliverables, services, products, or the like to be exchanged or provided.

Connecting for Health: A public-private collaborative that has representatives from more than 100 organizations across the spectrum of healthcare stakeholders. Its purpose is to catalyze the widespread changes necessary to realize the full benefits of health information technology (HIT), while protecting patient privacy and the security of personal health information. Connecting for Health is led and operated by the Markle Foundation with additional financial support from the Robert Wood Johnson Foundation. www.connectingforhealth.org

Continuity of Care Document (CCD): A specification that is an XML-based markup standard intended to specify the encoding, structure and semantics of a patient summary clinical document for exchange. The CCD specification is a constraint on the HL7 Clinical Document Architecture (CDA) standard and contains U.S. specific requirements; its use is therefore limited to the U.S.

Data set: A data repository or specifically defined collection of data, such as a health care record, electronic health record, claims record, or research data.

Data Use and Reciprocal Support Agreement (DURSA): A comprehensive, multi-party trust agreement that will be signed by all NHIN Health Information Exchanges (NHIEs), both public and private, wishing to participate in the Nationwide Health Information Network. The DURSA provides the legal framework governing participation in the NHIN by requiring the signatories to abide by a common set of terms and conditions. These common terms and conditions support the secure, interoperable exchange of health data between and among numerous NHIEs across the country.[3]

De-identified health information: De-identified health information consists of individual health records with data redacted or edited to prevent it from being associated with a specific individual. See the HIPAA Privacy Rule for de-identification guidelines. The term is defined at 45 C.F.R. § 160.103.[2]

EHR-Lab Interoperability and Connectivity Specification (ELINCS): Originally sponsored and developed by the California Healthcare Foundation (CHCF), ELINCS standardizes the formatting and coding of electronic messages exchanged between clinical laboratories and ambulatory electronic health record (EHR) systems. In 2008, ELINCS was adopted by HL7, the internationally recognized standards development organization for health information. HL7 will assume the ongoing maintenance and further development of ELINCS. www.elincs.org

Electronic Healthcare Network Accreditation Commission (EHNAC): A federally recognized standards development organization and tax-exempt, 501(c)6 non-profit accrediting body designed to improve transactional quality, operational efficiency, and data security in healthcare. EHNAC's accreditation services help electronic health networks, payer networks, financial services firms, and e-Prescribing and other solution providers improve business processes and expand market opportunities. www.ehnac.org/

Electronic health record (EHR): An electronic record of health-related information on an individual that conforms to nationally recognized interoperability standards and that can be created, managed, and consulted by authorized clinicians and staff across more than one healthcare organization.[6]

Electronic medical record (EMR): An electronic record of health-related information on an individual that can be created, gathered, managed, and consulted by authorized clinicians and staff within one healthcare organization.[6]

Encryption: A mathematical formula used to "scramble" data so it cannot be viewed while at rest or in transit by unauthorized individuals.

Healthcare Information and Management Systems Society (HIMSS): A "comprehensive healthcare-stakeholder membership organization exclusively focused on providing global leadership for the optimal use of information technology (IT) and management systems for the betterment of healthcare."[5] HIMSS works to develop healthcare public policy and industry practices through its advocacy, educational, and professional development initiatives. www.himss.org

Health Informatics Technology Standards Panel (HITSP): A public-private partnership, sponsored by ANSI under a contract from ONC, that was dedicated to facilitating the harmonization of consensus-based standards necessary to enable the widespread interoperability of healthcare information in the United States. www.hitsp.org

Health Information Exchange (HIE): The electronic movement of health-related information among organizations according to nationally recognized standards.[1] This term is interchangeable with HIO (Health Information Organization).

Health Information Organization (HIO): An organization that oversees and governs the exchange of health-related information among organizations according to nationally recognized standards.[6]

Health Information Technology for Economic and Clinical Health Act (HITECH Act): A bill that accomplishes four major goals that advance the use of health information technology: develop standards by 2010 that allow for the nationwide electronic exchange and use of health information to improve quality and coordination of care; invest $20 billion in health information technology infrastructure and Medicare and Medicaid incentives to encourage doctors and hospitals to use HIT to electronically exchange patients' health information; save the government $10 billion, and generate additional savings throughout the health sector, through improvements in quality of care and care coordination, and reductions in medical errors and duplicative care; strengthen federal privacy and security law to protect identifiable health information from misuse as the healthcare sector increases use of Health IT.

The Health Insurance Portability and Accountability Act of 1996 (HIPAA): HIPAA, specifically the HIPAA Administrative Simplification Provisions, includes the Privacy and Security Rules. HIPAA's Administrative Simplification Provisions required the U.S. Department of Health & Human Services (HHS) to adopt national standards for electronic health care transactions. At the same time, Congress recognized that advances in electronic technology could erode the privacy of health information. Consequently, Congress incorporated into HIPAA provisions that mandated the adoption of federal privacy protections for individually identifiable health information. HIPAA can be found at 45 CFR part 160, 45 CFR part 162, and 45 CFR part 164.[7]

Health Level Seven (HL7): An organization that develops standards for interoperability of health information technology. They are one of several ANSI-accredited standards-developing organizations operating in the healthcare arena. HL7's domain is clinical and administrative data. www.hl7.org

HHS: See **United States Department of Health & Human Services**

Integrating the Healthcare Enterprise (IHE): An organization that enables all stakeholders (users and developers) of healthcare information technology to achieve interoperability of systems leveraging standards and related standards-based operating rules and communications. www.ihe.net

Individually identifiable health information: As defined at 45 C.F.R § 160.103, "information that is a subset of health information, including demographic information collected from an individual, and: (1) Is created or received by a health care provider, health plan, employer, or health care clearinghouse; and (2) Relates to the past, present, or future physical or mental health or condition of an individual; the provision of health care to an individual; or the past, present, or future payment for the provision of health care to an individual; and (i) That identifies the individual; or (ii) With respect to which there is a reasonable basis to believe the information can be used to identify the individual."[2]

Information use and disclosure policies: Policies that define which data can be disclosed, what the data can be used for, and to whom the data can be disclosed. HIPAA defines allowable uses and disclosures of protected health information (PHI) at 45 C.F.R. § 164.502. However, non-covered entities are not bound by these restrictions.[8]

Logical Observation Identifiers Names and Codes (LOINC): Housed in the Regenstrief Institute, an internationally respected non-profit medical research organization associated with Indiana University, LOINC was developed by Regenstrief and the LOINC committee as a response to the demand for electronic movement of clinical data from laboratories that produce the data to hospitals, physician's offices, and payers who use the data for clinical care and management purposes. The purpose of LOINC® is to facilitate the exchange and pooling of clinical results for clinical care, outcomes management, and research by providing a set of universal codes and names to identify laboratory and other clinical observations. http://loinc.org/

National Committee on Vital and Health Statistics (NCVHS): A congressionally established advisory body to HHS. NCVHS advises HHS on the issues of health data, statistics, and national health information policy. In addition, NCVHS sponsors the Workgroup on National Health Information Infrastructure and Subcommittees on Privacy and Standards and Security. Recent recommendations to the secretary of HHS have included recommendations for the National Provider Identifier, integration for the Family Educational Rights and Privacy Act, and HIPAA. http://www.ncvhs.hhs.gov/

National Governors Association (NGA): "NGA provides governors and their senior staff members with services that range from representing states on Capitol Hill and before the Administration on key federal issues to developing policy reports on innovative state programs and hosting networking seminars for state government executive branch officials. The NGA Center for Best Practices focuses on state innovations and best practices on issues that range from education and health to technology, welfare reform, and the environment. NGA also provides management and technical assistance to both new and incumbent governors."[9] www.nga.org (Also see **State Alliance for e-Health.**)

Nationwide Health Information Network (NHIN): A "set of standards, services, and policies that enable secure health information exchange over the Internet. The NHIN will provide a foundation for the exchange of health IT across diverse entities, within communities and across the country, helping to achieve the goals of the HITECH Act. This critical part of the national health IT agenda will enable health information to follow the consumer, be available for clinical decision making, and support appropriate use of healthcare information beyond direct patient care so as to improve population health."[10]

Network: (1) More than one computer, generally connected to a server, supporting an organization's information technology operations. (2) "A collection of hardware, such as printers, modems, servers, and terminals/personal computers that enables users to store and retrieve information, share devices, and exchange information."[1]

Object Management Group (OMG): An international, open membership, not-for-profit computer industry consortium. OMG Task Forces develop enterprise integration standards for a wide range of technologies and an even wider range of industries. www.omg.org/

Office of the National Coordinator for Health Information Technology (ONC): Organizationally located within the Office of the Secretary for the U.S. Department of Health & Human Services (HHS) and is at the forefront of the administration's health IT efforts as a resource to the entire health system to support the adoption of health information technology and the promotion of nationwide health information exchange to improve healthcare. www.healthit.hhs.gov/portal/server.pt

Personal health record (PHR): An electronic record of health-related information on an individual that conforms to nationally recognized interoperability standards and that can be drawn from multiple sources while being managed, shared, and controlled by the individual.[6]

Policy: (1) High-level statement of an organization's approach to security, privacy, and other business-related practices. (2) "Overall intention and direction as formally expressed by management."[1]

Procedure: Specifically defines how a policy is to be implemented within an organization and the steps required to adhere to established policy.

Protected health information (PHI): Individually identifiable health data specifically protected under the HIPAA Privacy and Security Rules. The same information held by a non-covered entity is not PHI. The term is defined at 45 C.F.R. § 164.501, and additional information on uses and disclosures of PHI can be found at 45 C.F.R. § 164.502.[8]

Provider: (1) An individual or group of individuals who directly (primary care physicians, psychiatrists, nurses, surgeons, etc.) or indirectly (laboratories, radiology clinics, etc) provide healthcare to patients. (2) Any supplier of a healthcare service.[1]

Regulatory agencies: Agencies of the government that often report to the executive branch (state and federal). They regulate the activity of organizations and individuals as generally outlined in rules or regulations (e.g., Medicaid agencies, public health authorities, Board of Medical Examiners, insurance commissions, consumer protection agencies).

Request for proposal (RFP): A request for proposals from vendors to perform a scope of work defined by the contracting entity.

Regional Health Information Organization (RHIO): An organization formed to exchange information for the purposes of improving quality of care, efficiency, or safety. The term RHIO is often used interchangeably with the terms HIE or HIO.

Stakeholder: Any organization or individual that has a stake in the exchange of health information, including healthcare providers, health plans, healthcare clearinghouses, regulatory agencies, associations, consumers, and technology vendors.

State Alliance for e-Health: An NGA-led initiative, funded by ONC, designed to improve the nation's healthcare system through the formation of a collaborative body that enables states to increase the efficiency and effectiveness of the HIT initiatives they develop. The State Alliance provides a nationwide forum through which stakeholders can work together to identify interstate- and intrastate-based HIT policies and best practices and explore solutions to programmatic and legal issues related to the exchange of health information. www.nga.org/portal/site/nga/menuitem.1f41d49be2d3d33eacdcbeeb501010a0/ ?vgnextoid=5066b5bd2b991110VgnVCM1000001a01010aRCRD

Systematized Nomenclature of Medicine - Clinical Terms (SNOMED-CT): A comprehensive, multilingual clinical healthcare terminology coding system supported by the International Health Terminology Standards Development Organization (IHTSD), an international not-for-profit organization based in Denmark. www.ihtsdo. org/snomed-ct/

United States Department of Health & Human Services (HHS): The United States government's principal agency for protecting the health of all Americans and providing essential human services, especially for those who are least able to help themselves. www.hhs.gov

Workgroup for Electronic Data Interchange (WEDI): Established in 1991 in response to a challenge from then-Secretary of Health & Human Services, Louis Sullivan, MD. The challenge was to bring together a consortium of leaders within the healthcare industry to identify practical strategies for reducing administrative costs in healthcare through the implementation of EDI. WEDI quickly became a major advocate in promoting the acceptance and implementation of the standardization of administrative and financial healthcare data. WEDI's goal is "to provide multi-stakeholder leadership and guidance to the healthcare industry on how to use and leverage the industry's collective knowledge, expertise, and information resources to improve the quality, affordability, and availability of healthcare." WEDI provides information on HIPAA and has a Privacy Policy Advisory Group.[11] www.wedi.org

REFERENCES

1. HIMSS. *HIMSS Dictionary of Healthcare Information Technology Terms, Acronyms and Organizations, Second Edition.* Chicago: HIMSS; 2010.

2. *Code of Federal Regulations, Title 45, Part 160 – General Administrative Requirements, Section 103 - Definitions.* US Government Printing Office; 2009.

3. NHIN Cooperative DURSA Workgroup. Data Use and Reciprocal Support Agreement (DURSA). Posted January 23, 2009. http://healthit.hhs.gov/portal/server.pt/gateway/PTARGS_0_10731_ 849891_0_0_18/DRAFT%20NHIN%20Trial%20Implementations%20Production%20DURSA-3.pdf. Accessed April 7, 2010.

4. HIMSS – About HIMSS. http://www.himss.org/ASP/aboutHimssHome.asp. Accessed April 7, 2010.

5. Department of Health & Human Services, Office of the National Coordinator for Health Information Technology. Defining Key Health Information Technology Terms. Posted April 28, 2008. http://healthit.hhs.gov/portal/server.pt/gateway/PTARGS_0_10741_848133_0_0_18/10_2_hit_terms.pdf. Accessed April 7, 2010.

6. *Code of Federal Regulations, Title 45 – Public Welfare.* US Government Printing Office; 2009.

7. *Code of Federal Regulations, Title 45, Part 164 – Security and Privacy.* US Government Printing Office; 2009.

8. NGA – About the National Governors Association. http://www.nga.org/portal/site/nga/menuitem.cdd492add7dd9cf9e8ebb856a11010a0/. Accessed April 7, 2010

9. HHS - ONC Initiatives - Nationwide Health Information Network (NHIN): Overview. http://healthit.hhs.gov/portal/server.pt?open=512&mode=2&cached=true&objID=1142. Accessed April 7, 2010.

10. WEDI. www.wedi.org. Accessed April 7, 2010.

Index

H

I